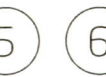
CW01501057

Contents

(10)

Summary

- Sustainability and transformation plans (STPs) are plans for the future of health and care services in England. NHS organisations in different parts of the country have been asked to collaborate to respond to the challenges facing local services. This marks a decisive shift from the focus on competition as a means of improving health service performance in the Health and Social Care Act 2012.

- Our research focused on how STPs are being developed in different parts of the country, based on interviews with senior NHS and local government leaders in four STP areas. While leaders supported the idea of working together to improve services and manage limited resources, the process of developing STPs has been challenging.

- It is important to recognise the context in which the plans are being developed. The pressures facing local services are significant and growing, and the timescales available to develop the plans have been extremely tight. The plans are also being developed within the fragmented and complex organisational arrangements created by the Health and Social Care Act. In this context, credit needs to be given to local areas for the progress made on STPs so far, notwithstanding the major challenges identified in this report.

- The start of the STP process was characterised by a high level of intervention from NHS England and NHS Improvement in defining geographical boundaries for the plans and identifying STP leaders. The national requirements and deadlines have been ambiguous and have changed over time. Guidance for STP areas on the detail of the plans has often arrived later than promised or, in some cases, did not arrive at all. The approaches of national NHS bodies and their regional teams have not always been consistent.

- The original purpose of STPs was to support local areas to improve care quality and efficiency of services, develop new models of care, and prioritise prevention and public health. The emphasis from national NHS bodies has shifted over time to focus more heavily on how STPs can bring the NHS into financial balance (quickly). National NHS leaders are themselves under

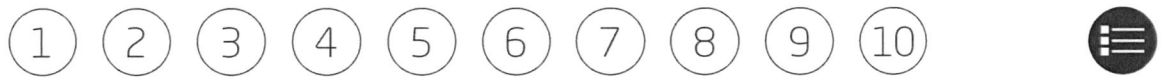

pressure from central government to close gaps in NHS finances, at a time when the NHS faces an unprecedented slowdown in funding and dramatic cuts have been made to public health and social care budgets. It is therefore important to recognise the constraints facing national as well as local leaders in the NHS.

- STP leaders and teams have worked hard to develop their plans on top of their existing day jobs and various other initiatives. This has not been easy. The additional workload for most areas has been significant and is unlikely to be sustainable in the long term. Management consultants are also routinely being used to support the local STP process.

- The limited time available to develop STPs has made it difficult for local leaders to meaningfully involve all parts of the health and care system – particularly clinicians and frontline staff – in developing the plans. The involvement of local authorities has varied widely between STP areas, ranging from strong partnership between the NHS and local government to almost no local government involvement at all. Patients and the public have been largely absent from the STP process so far.

- Progress made on the plans in different areas is highly dependent on local context and the history of collaboration across the STP area. Where good relationships already existed, these provided a positive foundation for joint working on the STP. Some areas were able to draw on pre-existing plans for service changes to take forward in their STP, and have made progress in developing a sense of 'common purpose' between leaders. Where relationships were poor, securing engagement in the process was a challenge in itself. The geographical context and the complexity of the system have also been important factors.

- As well as practical challenges to developing STPs, leaders faced fundamental policy barriers to working together and making collective decisions. STPs are being developed in an environment that was not designed to support collaboration between organisations. In particular, our research highlighted the significant policy gap between existing accountability arrangements in the NHS – focused on individual organisations – and the kind of collective governance arrangements needed for STPs to function. The national approach to regulation and performance management in the NHS reinforces this tension.

- The focus of the STP process so far has been on planning. But leaders in all areas were concerned about their ability to implement their plans in practice. Doing this will require a different set of skills, resources and approaches by local leaders. It will also require a greater focus on the relational and cultural processes of managing change.

- We make a number of recommendations for the future of the STP process based on our findings. At a local level, involvement in the process needs to be strengthened and more robust governance and leadership arrangements developed to allow for collective decision-making between organisations. This in turn will require action from national bodies in the NHS to remove the policy barriers that get in the way of joint working and provide guidance on how organisations can pool sovereignty in practice.

- There is a need for more co-ordinated leadership at national level to avoid the fragmentation experienced throughout the process so far. Given the speed at which STPs have been developed, the plans and the analysis underpinning them will require 'stress-testing' to ensure that the financial assumptions they make are sound and the service changes they propose can be delivered.

- If this can be done, collective action through STPs offers an important opportunity for improving health and care services in England. In many ways, STPs are a complex 'workaround' to the existing NHS structures and legislation that pull the system away from collaboration. Making STPs work in practice will therefore require time and effort from NHS staff and leaders at all levels, who will inevitably face challenges as the process continues. There have been significant issues with the STP process so far. But place-based working is by far a preferable alternative to the 'fortress mentality' whereby NHS organisations act to secure their own future regardless of the impact on others.

Introduction

Sustainability and transformation plans (STPs) were introduced in NHS planning guidance published in December 2015 (NHS England *et al* 2015). NHS organisations in different parts of England were asked to come together to develop plans for the future of health services in their area, including by working with local authorities and other partners. These plans are being called STPs. Forty-four areas were identified as the geographical 'footprints' on which the plans would be based, and final plans were due to be completed in October 2016.

STPs represent a significant and wide-reaching exercise in health care planning in England, covering all areas of NHS spending on services from 2016/17 to 2020/21. They also represent an important shift in NHS policy on improvement and reform. While the Health and Social Care Act 2012 sought to strengthen the role of competition within the health care system, NHS organisations are now being told to collaborate rather than compete to plan and provide local services (Alderwick and Ham 2016). This is being called 'place-based planning'.

Given the history of short-term policy initiatives in the NHS and the speed at which new initiatives are often introduced (Ham 2014), the future of STPs is by no means certain. But they look like they are here to stay for now, at least. Recent operational planning and contracting guidance for the NHS sought to further embed STPs into NHS planning processes over the next two years (NHS England and NHS Improvement 2016a).

STPs have attracted growing media attention since they were first announced (*see* box, pp 14–5), particularly after some draft plans were published following an early planning deadline in June 2016. Major service changes are being considered in many of the plans (Edwards 2016), often involving changes to acute hospital services, and cautions have been raised about the kind of benefits that these changes can deliver (Murray *et al* 2016a).

The plans have also attracted growing political attention. A large number of parliamentary questions have been asked about STPs since June 2016 (*see* Appendix). The plans were the subject of an opposition day debate in the House of Commons in September 2016, when many Members of Parliament (MPs) voiced concerns about potential cuts to services and the 'secrecy' of the STP process (Hansard (House of Commons Debates) 2016–17). Questions about STPs have also been raised at the Public Accounts Committee (House of Commons Public Accounts Committee 2016) and the Health Select Committee (House of Commons Health Committee 2016).

Despite the importance of STPs for the NHS and the public, little is known about the process of developing the plans and how the initiative has worked in practice. The purpose of this qualitative study was to understand how STPs are being developed in different parts of the country and to identify lessons that can be learnt for local areas and national policy-makers.

Specifically, we wanted to understand:

- how the work to develop STPs was being led, governed and managed at a local level

- the extent of collaboration in developing STPs and the involvement of different partners

- the role of external advice and support in developing STPs – for example, by management consultants

- how the process has been managed at a national level and the relationship between national bodies in the NHS and local areas

- how the process was perceived by local leaders and the challenges experienced in developing STPs.

To do this, we carried out a series of interviews with senior NHS and local government leaders involved in developing STPs in four parts of the country. This report is based on analysis of data from these interviews. It therefore focuses on the local experience and perceptions of the STP process by those directly involved in developing the plans. Taken together, the four STP areas involved in the study cover a combined population of around 5 million people – just under 10 per cent of the total population of England.

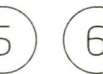

Methods

We selected the four areas using criteria to ensure that we chose a relatively representative sample of STP areas. The criteria included considerations about geographical location and characteristics, STP leadership, and the history of collaboration between organisations in the area. We selected one STP area from each of NHS England's four regions. We then identified between seven and ten senior leaders involved in developing the STP in each of these four areas to take part in interviews. Again, we used criteria to ensure that these leaders represented different parts of the health and care system. In each STP area, this included leaders from NHS providers and commissioners, local government, NHS England's regional team, and representatives from the team managing day-to-day work on the STP.

We interviewed the same group of leaders (unless staff had moved on or changed roles, in which case we interviewed a replacement) at two points in the STP process: first, in April 2016, and then again, in June and July 2016. We carried out a total of 56 semi-structured interviews with 32 people. Interviews were recorded and transcribed. We conducted a thematic analysis of the interviews and summary notes using NVivo (computer software to support qualitative analysis). The four STP areas and the leaders involved in our research are anonymised in this report. We sometimes use the blanket term 'leaders' to describe our interviewees throughout the paper.

Structure of the report

The report comprises three parts. The first (Section 2) sets out the background and context of STPs, including a timeline of the STP process and the scope of the plans. The second (Sections 3 to 8) describes the findings from our research, covering the key themes and details from our interviews with local leaders. The final part (Sections 9 and 10) explores the implications of our findings and makes recommendations for the future of the STP process.

This report is the first of two papers that The King's Fund will publish describing the findings of our research into the development of STPs. The second paper will focus on the content and implementation of the plans and will be based on interviews with the same group of leaders, carried out from September to November 2016, and analysis of other data.

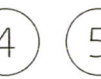   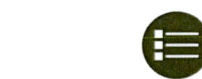

② Background and context

In October 2014, NHS England and other national bodies published the *NHS five year forward view* (Forward View). The Forward View set out a vision of how NHS services need to change in future to meet the needs of the population. It argued that the NHS needed to place far greater emphasis on prevention, integration of services, and putting people in control of their own health. It described the 'new care models' needed to make these changes happen, based on collaboration between different parts of the health and care system. Putting in place these new care models was seen as one way to address the growing gaps in NHS finances.

The aim of STPs is to support the NHS to deliver the changes set out in the Forward View. At their most simple, STPs are plans for the future of health and care services across defined geographical areas in England (such as Somerset or Derbyshire). They were introduced in NHS planning guidance published in December 2015, which asked local NHS organisations to come together to develop 'place-based' plans for how services will be delivered in their area – centred on local populations rather than individual organisations. The plans needed to cover all areas of NHS spending, including specialised services and primary care, as well as focusing on better integration with social care and other local authority services. They also needed to be long term, covering the period from October 2016 to March 2021.

The initial guidance outlined around 60 questions for local areas to consider in their plans, covering three headline areas: improving quality and developing new models of care; improving health and wellbeing; and improving efficiency of services. Local leaders were also asked to show how their plans would deliver financial balance for the NHS in their area – a theme that has become more prominent as the planning process has gone on.

While the plans themselves are clearly important, the guidance emphasised that STPs are about more than just 'writing a document'. Instead, they needed to be based on:

- local leaders coming together as a team
- developing a shared vision with the local community (including local government)

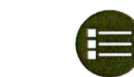

- planning a coherent set of activities to make the vision happen

- delivering the plan

- learning and adapting as the process goes on.

Early in 2016, 44 parts of the country were identified as the geographical areas on which the plans would be based – referred to as STP 'footprints'. The average footprint covers 1.2 million people, but their size varies significantly: the smallest covers 300,000 people and the largest covers 2.8 million (NHS England 2016h). Each STP footprint spans an average of five clinical commissioning group (CCG) areas but, again, the number of organisations involved varies widely: some footprints cover only one CCG area and others cover as many as 12 CCGs. Many more NHS providers and other organisations exist within each footprint. A named individual was chosen to lead the development of each STP. The process for identifying STP footprints and leaders is explored in Section 3.

The timelines for developing STPs and the process for approving them have been somewhat fluid. The original deadline for submitting plans to NHS England and other national bodies was the end of June 2016. But this deadline was pushed back to the end of October 2016 – with the June plans reframed as initial drafts. Additional planning requirements have also been added as the process has gone on. Table 1 provides a timeline of the STP process from December 2015 to October 2016 – including key announcements, guidance, deadlines and events related to the plans. A more detailed timeline is included in the Appendix.

Once the final STPs were submitted in October 2016, it was intended that they would be assessed by national NHS bodies. The plans were to be agreed and used to form the basis of new operational plans for NHS organisations and contracts between commissioners and providers (NHS England and NHS Improvement 2016a). It is currently unclear what will happen in areas where STPs are not agreed by national bodies, and – at the time of writing – it is likely that a number of STP areas will not be able to submit plans that have been fully 'signed-off' by local leaders. Access to additional funding for the NHS announced in the 2015 Spending Review will be linked to the quality of the plans that are submitted; from April 2017, STPs will become the single application and approval process for accessing NHS transformation funding, with the best plans set to receive funds soonest.

Table 1 STP process timeline summary

Guidance, announcement or planning deadline	Date	Key points
National NHS bodies publish shared planning guidance for the NHS (NHS England *et al* 2015)	22 December 2015	Asks NHS leaders to come together in geographical footprints (to be signed off by national bodies) to produce STPs by the end of June 2016
Monitor publishes research (Monitor 2015a)	24 December 2015	To help organisations think about their STP footprints
Deadline for localities to submit proposals for STP footprints	29 January 2016	
Letter from national NHS bodies on STP guidance (NHS England 2016b)	16 February 2016	Invites footprints to nominate a leader to oversee their STP
Letter from Chair of Local Government Association (LGA) to Secretary of State for Health (Seccombe 2016)	10 March 2016	Expresses 'concern' about pace of implementation and lack of involvement of local councils
44 geographical footprints announced (NHS England 2016h)	15 March 2016	
STP leaders announced (in all but three areas) (NHS England 2016g)	30 March 2016	Leaders are mainly from CCGs and NHS trusts or foundation trusts, but three are from local government (a fourth leader from local government is announced subsequently)
April STP checkpoint (NHS England 2016a)	15 April 2016	Initial STP submission to set out early thinking on the plan
One-to-one meetings with senior representatives from national NHS bodies to discuss April submissions	April/May 2016	
Guidance on June submission (NHS England 2016f)	18 May 2016	June deadline for full STPs is now a 'checkpoint' for draft plans, which should include details of '3–5 critical decisions' needed by 2020/21
Indicative funds to 2020 published (NHS England 2016c)	19 May 2016	Setting out indicative funding for STP footprints to 2020/21
'Quick guides' for STPs published (NHS England 2016d)	19 May 2016	Covering 14 topics, to help STPs tackle local system challenges
Finance template sent to STP leads (NHS Improvement 2016d)	1 June 2016	Each footprint to 'show how it will close its financial gap' by 2020/21

continued on next page

Table 1 STP process timeline summary *continued*

Guidance, announcement or planning deadline	Date	Key points
NHS Confederation annual conference	17 June 2016	The topic of STPs is covered by many speakers: • Simon Stevens, Chief Executive of NHS England, suggests that in some places local authorities may take on more of a leadership role for NHS functions • Jeremy Hunt, Secretary of State for Health, says that 'The STPs are very simply about reducing hospital bed days... and reducing emergency admissions'
Letter from Jim Mackey and Ed Smith about 2016/17 financial position (NHS England and NHS Improvement 2016b, Annex C)	28 June 2016	Announces further action to reduce deficits, with STP leads asked to identify 'unsustainable' services by 31 July 2016
June 'checkpoint'	30 June 2016	STP leaders submit draft plans, to be discussed with leaders of national NHS bodies in July 2016
Senior leaders within national NHS bodies visit all 44 STP areas	July 2016	Conversations held between each of the 44 footprints and national NHS teams to review draft STP submissions
Financial reset (NHS England and NHS Improvement 2016b)	21 July 2016	Access to 2016/17 Sustainability and Transformation Fund 'assumes full and effective participation' by providers in STPs. CCG funding allocation growth in 2017/18 conditional on national approval of STP
Update from NHS England and NHS Improvement on June submissions (West 2016)	19 August 2016	Letters to each STP warn of an 'extremely constrained capital environment', suggest system control totals to be made available to advanced STPs, and set deadline of 21 October 2016 for submission of full STPs
NHS Improvement publishes single oversight framework for NHS providers (NHS Improvement 2016c)	13 September 2016	Providers to be assessed on range of areas, including 'strategic change', with a particular focus on contribution to STPs
An opposition day debate on STPs is held in the House of Commons	14 September 2016	Shadow Health Secretary Diane Abbott MP proposes a motion stating 'concern' about STPs, which may 'lead to significant cuts' and lack transparency. The House votes against the motion
NHS England publishes guidance for involving patients and communities (NHS England 2016k)	15 September 2016	Suggests most areas will publish their plans between October 2016 and the end of the year

continued on next page

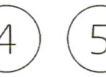

Table 1 **STP process timeline summary** *continued*

Guidance, announcement or planning deadline	Date	Key points
NHS England and NHS Improvement publish shared planning guidance for 2017–19 (NHS England and NHS Improvement 2016a)	22 September 2016	Guidance covers two financial years. From April 2017, each STP area is to be given a shared financial control total. Announces that baseline metrics for STPs will be published in November 2016
Deadline for final STP submissions	21 October 2016	

Media coverage of sustainability and transformation plans

We tracked* print and online media coverage of STPs from December 2015 to September 2016. We focused on news stories about the plans and were interested in changes in focus and volume of stories over time.

In the early stages of the process, coverage about STPs was limited to news items in trade publications (such as the *Health Service Journal*). But once STP footprints were announced in March, STPs started to gain wider media attention – particularly from regional news outlets, which reported on local appointments to STP leadership roles.

The volume of regional media activity increased in April. References to STPs appeared in news items about the 'financial crisis' facing NHS services, alongside terms such as 'privatisation', 'radical restructuring' and 'fear'.

The concept of winners and losers in STPs entered regional media reports in May. Some stories reported concerns that rural areas could 'lose out' as a result of the plans. Articles also reported that a range of stakeholders (including GPs and local authorities) felt 'shut out' of the STP process.

National media interest in STPs began in June, in response to comments about the financial challenges facing the NHS made by speakers at the NHS Confederation's annual conference.

continued on next page

*We searched national newspaper websites and Google news to identify relevant stories.

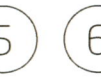

Media coverage of sustainability and transformation plans *continued*

The role of local authorities in the plans dominated media activity in July. The chief executive of Warrington Borough Council, for example, was reported describing STPs as 'arrogant' and a 'recipe for disaster' (Everett 2016). At the same time, several stories appeared in regional media reporting on the potential benefits of STPs, including 'improved health' and 'reduced waiting times'.

In late July and early August, the tone of media coverage became more negative. The volume of coverage also increased. On 26 August, the campaigning group 38 Degrees published an investigation into STPs that was covered by all major newspaper and broadcast outlets. News items focused on the 'secrecy' and lack of public consultation on the plans, as well as making frequent links to potential 'cuts', ward closures and the downgrading of A&E services.

September was the busiest month for regional media on STPs. Articles focused on what STPs might mean for particular services in different parts of the country, after some draft plans were 'leaked' into the public domain. These articles were typically concerned with NHS services and beds being 'axed', 'centralised' and 'closed'. Coverage also continued in national broadsheets – although their focus was less on service changes and more on the secrecy of the process. Some pieces linked STPs to the possible privatisation of the NHS.

Media coverage of STPs seems set to continue, and is likely to grow once the final plans are published.

Why do STPs matter?

The NHS in England faces significant financial and service pressures. NHS provider deficits reached an all-time high of £2.45 billion in 2015/16. Additional funding has been used to try to fill these deficits, but it has not removed them entirely – and the gap between demand for services and available funding continues to grow. Key performance targets are being missed all year round, general practice is in crisis, and community and mental health services are under huge pressure (Murray *et al* 2016b). The crisis in social care services is perhaps even more severe (Humphries *et al* 2016). As well as meeting these day-to-day pressures, NHS staff are in the process of redesigning services to better meet the needs of the population.

The NHS is trying to meet these challenges in the context of the Health and Social Care Act and its legacy of fragmented and complex organisational arrangements (Ham *et al* 2015). The Act strengthened the role of competition within the NHS and created uncertainties about when services should be put out to tender. Commissioning responsibilities were fragmented between a number of organisations, both within the NHS and between the NHS and local government. And the abolition of strategic health authorities (SHAs) created a vacuum in system leadership in the NHS at a local level, making it difficult to co-ordinate improvements in care between large numbers of commissioners and providers of services.

The introduction of STPs reflects a growing consensus that more co-ordinated action is needed to meet the challenges facing the NHS and social care services. Growing numbers of people living with complex health needs, for example, require care that is co-ordinated both within the NHS and between the NHS and social care (Naylor *et al* 2016; Oliver *et al* 2014). Collaboration is also needed to address the wider social, economic and environmental determinants of health across society. This means NHS organisations working closely with other services and sectors to focus on the broader aim of improving population health – not just delivering better and more sustainable health care (Alderwick *et al* 2015a).

Dealing with growing financial deficits in the NHS also requires a systemic response, avoiding the 'tragedy of the commons' that is all too apparent in the NHS today (Dunn *et al* 2016; Ham and Alderwick 2015). The same is true between the NHS and local government, as the pressures facing NHS and social care services (and their impact on the population) are closely linked (Humphries *et al* 2016).

STPs therefore offer an important opportunity for NHS and local government leaders to work together to address the collective challenges facing their local populations. Whether or not these ambitions can be achieved, however, is yet to be seen. STPs stand in a long line of planning initiatives in the NHS that have tried to bring together different organisations to improve services. In 2013, for instance, CCGs and their partners (including NHS providers and local government) were asked to develop five-year plans to transform services and prioritise prevention (NHS England and Public Health England 2013). These plans have since been largely forgotten. The same experience is true right across the public sector. Over the past two decades, a raft of public policy initiatives has been introduced in England with the aim of 'joining up' services at a local level – but success stories, while they exist, are hard to find (Wilson *et al* 2015). Will things be any different this time around? The process of how STPs are being developed – explored in this report – is likely to play a major part in answering this question.

❸ How was the STP process set up?

Before areas could begin work on their STPs, decisions needed to be taken about the geographical boundaries of each plan and who would be responsible for leading them. The process for making these decisions varied between areas, affecting both how the plans progressed and leaders' perceptions of the STP process. In this section we describe how these decisions were taken and outline the types of governance arrangements that were put in place to oversee the development of the plans.

Defining STP boundaries

One of the first tasks of the STP process was to define the geographical areas to be covered by each plan – referred to as STP 'footprints'. Planning guidance asked local leaders to make proposals for their STP footprints by the end of January 2016. All areas in England needed to be covered by a footprint, which the guidance suggested should be 'larger rather than smaller' to meet the challenges facing local services. The footprints were to be 'locally defined' as a result of engagement between NHS and local government leaders.

Taken together, STP footprints in our four areas emerged through a combination of top-down direction from national NHS bodies and bottom-up agreement by local leaders. For two of our areas, the footprints were primarily defined by local leaders, based on the geographical boundaries of existing NHS initiatives or well-established organisational boundaries. While local authority leaders did not always feel included in decisions to establish these boundaries, the STP footprints in these two areas seemed to broadly 'make sense' to most NHS leaders.

In our other two areas, national NHS bodies played a much greater role in defining the STP footprints. Local leaders made initial proposals for multiple STPs to be developed in their area – again, based on existing initiatives and what they perceived to be natural population groupings and patient flows. But these proposals were not accepted by the national bodies, who wanted organisations in both places to work together across larger geographical areas. This meant national NHS bodies directly intervening to overrule the plans of local leaders and bring together two or three areas into a larger STP footprint:

> *Then the regulators got involved and we were effectively told that… I'm being really frank and open… We were told that the number was wrong, so there were too many STP footprints in our region, and the number had to be reduced, and therefore [place X] rather than having two should have one.*

> *I think we were told what our footprint needed to be if I was perfectly honest.*

> *Basically they were told: no, you need to have one footprint across [place X].*

The nature of this intervention caused some tensions between local leaders, who often felt that they had been forced to work together across a footprint that made little sense to their local population or their own organisation. Concerns were raised that work on the STP would hold back existing plans for collaboration at a more local level. Leaders also described the challenge of understanding how their local priorities would fit within a broader STP, and which issues should be addressed at what geographical level.

For leaders in local government, the STP footprints did not always fit with their own plans and priorities. For example, the STP footprints sometimes conflicted with boundaries already agreed within local government for devolution plans. In one area, a devolution plan being developed by local government spanned two STP footprints. In another area, two devolution plans sit within a single STP footprint. Some local government leaders also told us they had no meaningful involvement in helping define the STP footprint in the first place. One, for instance, told us that the footprint was 'fundamentally defined by the NHS. And we were advised and told about it and that was about it.'

Similar boundary challenges also existed for some NHS providers. Across the four areas involved in our research, there were examples of acute, community, mental health and ambulance services provided by one organisation but split between more than one STP. This caused difficulties for planning purposes, with providers struggling to engage in the development of more than one plan. As one NHS provider chief executive told us: 'I don't think the centre thought through the implications of how organisations were supposed to try to keep engaged in all of those.' In one case, these problems are likely to lead to the redrawing of the STP boundary to more adequately account for patient flows and provider relationships.

Whichever way the footprints were defined, leaders from all areas talked about the various sub-systems that existed within their footprint – typically with two or three smaller and well-established geographical groupings making up their wider STP footprint. For many leaders, these smaller sub-systems held more meaning for planning purposes than the larger STP footprint they were now working in.

Identifying STP leaders

Each STP area was asked by national NHS bodies to select a named individual to lead the development of their plan. They were told that the individual should be 'a senior and credible leader who can command the trust and confidence of the system, such as a CCG Chief Officer, a provider Chief Executive or a Local Authority Chief Executive' (NHS England 2016b, Annex A). The process for doing this in our four areas varied, but was rarely seen as being open or fair.

We found that NHS England and NHS Improvement played a significant role in selecting STP leaders. In one area, the STP leader was nominated by NHS England's regional team rather than selected through a process of local discussion. In another area, local leaders had agreed their own candidate to lead the STP but were overruled by national bodies. An alternative candidate – another chief executive from the footprint – was appointed directly by a national leader in the NHS. In a third area, local leaders had decided to advertise for an independent STP leader from outside their area, but again found their decision overruled by national leaders. An alternative leader was imposed without local discussion.

The reasons offered by local leaders for this intervention varied. Some felt that national bodies in the NHS wanted to achieve a fixed distribution of STP leaders from different kinds of organisations, so intervened in some areas to even the balance (say, towards NHS provider chief executives). Some felt that it was because national leaders preferred particular leadership styles over others – for instance,

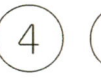

wanting 'somebody who could knock some heads together and get some things done'. For others, it was a combination of factors.

While local leaders were often (but not always) content with the STP leader who had been imposed on them from above, the nature of this intervention caused significant tensions at a local level, as well as feelings of unfairness and mistrust in the STP process more broadly. This in turn had an impact on local leaders' perceptions of their own ability to make change happen. One leader, for example, told us how the intervention made them feel 'impotent' – like 'we have no control over our own destiny'. Another said:

> It's not about [leader X], it's about the process. There's a massive cultural shift that is going to have to happen, and that won't happen if then ultimately [organisation X] turns around and says 'actually, this is what's happening'. For this change/transformation to really manifest and be able to be embedded, there's a huge amount of trust that has to be there, and has to be there across the leaders in order for them to model it. If we don't trust what's going on we're not going to be able to model that with our own workforces and engage them in the change.

The strong role played by national bodies also seemed at odds with the original emphasis on the STP process being locally led:

> So on the one hand, we had a policy emerging where local communities were meant to develop their own approach and leadership, and then from the top down came 'no, you're having X'.

The experience was different in only one of our four areas, where the STP leader emerged through a process of local discussion, negotiation and agreement. This included discussion at a system leadership group meeting involving representatives from both the NHS and local government, as well as a number of individual conversations between leaders. In our other three areas, leaders from local government were largely absent from conversations about STP leadership – although the same was true for a range of leaders from within the NHS too.

Establishing governance and management arrangements

Once STP boundaries and leaders had been established, organisations in each area worked to put in place new governance arrangements to support the development of their STP. This primarily involved creating ways to:

- discuss issues and make decisions between senior leaders

- organise and co-ordinate work on the STP

- involve relevant partners at different stages in the process

- gain agreement on plans between different organisations.

In three of our four areas, leaders put in place a broadly similar set of arrangements to try to do this – albeit at different speeds. Pre-existing system leadership groups were adapted to become the senior leadership team for the STP. These groups typically involved chief executives from commissioners and large providers in the NHS, as well as representatives from local government. Programme management offices were established to undertake and co-ordinate work on the STP, along with working groups covering different themes (such as workforce or finance). These groups drew on existing work and staff where possible, as well as relying on support from management consultants (*see* Section 6).

In the fourth of our areas, leaders struggled to put in place governance arrangements to support the development of their STP. While work to develop the plan was being done by a small set of individuals from different parts of the system, it was not taking place within an agreed governance structure or programme of work. Leaders had considered merging work on the STP with an existing programme of work focused on the reconfiguration of acute hospital services in their area (based on the same geographical footprint as the STP), but this idea was rejected because of concerns that it would limit the focus of their STP to acute services. Proposals had been developed to establish a separate system leadership group to oversee work on the STP, but these plans had not been agreed and the group had not yet met at the time of our research.

Across all four areas, leaders talked about the need for work on the STP to feed into existing governance and decision-making processes in different parts of the local system, such as the meetings of NHS trust boards and health and wellbeing boards.

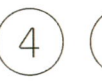 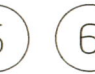

This was particularly important given that STP leaders and the various governance processes they created lacked any formal authority or decision-making powers (this point is explored further in Section 4).

The groups most obviously absent from STP governance processes were patients and the public. By the time of our second round of interviews (June and July 2016), none of the four areas had developed concrete plans to engage the public directly in the development of their STP. This was partly because of the limited time available to develop the plans, and partly because national NHS bodies had asked leaders to keep their draft STPs out of the public domain. This is explored in more detail in Section 5.

4 How have STPs been led and governed?

Putting in place leadership and governance arrangements is one thing, but making them work in practice is altogether more difficult. Leaders described a range of practical and policy challenges to working together on STPs and making decisions across organisations. The question of how STPs will be governed in future is being asked across all STP areas – but answers are proving difficult to find within existing policy and accountability arrangements in the NHS. This section of the paper explores these challenges. It also focuses on the overall leadership of STPs and what the role of STP leaders means in practice.

Practical challenges

In all STP areas it has been difficult to involve all relevant parts of the health and care system in the STP process – particularly key groups such as GPs, other clinicians and local authorities. The large number of organisations involved in commissioning and providing care in each STP area presented obvious challenges for securing widespread engagement in the process within the time available. Levels of involvement of different groups are described in Section 5. Where there was little history of collaboration across the STP footprint, this made the task of securing involvement in the STP more difficult. And in areas where the STP footprint had been imposed from above rather than defined locally, getting leaders and organisations to think as 'one footprint' rather than multiple planning areas was an added challenge.

When leaders from different organisations were able to come together to discuss work on the STP, the sheer number of organisations represented at STP meetings in most areas was often seen as a barrier to getting things done:

> *The amount of faces around a table… is what is hindering this whole process. It's like the Eurovision Song Contest at the moment: when you want to make a*

decision it goes around the table and by the time everybody says whether they've agreed it – yes or no – you've lost an hour. It's madness.

Whenever I go to a health meeting I'm sat at a table with 30 or more people, and a group of that size cannot make decisions in my opinion. I really do not envy them this task, because I don't think I would know how to do it….

Partly because of this, leaders typically felt that difficult decisions between organisations had not yet been taken as part of the STP process. The lack of detail in most draft plans – some described simply as 'a plan for a plan' – meant that 'big issues' had often been easy to avoid:

Well, the dynamic at the moment is it's all quite general. It's quite high level and it lacks specifically [and] we haven't really got into any issues which require decision essentially.

It's all… everybody's working together, it's all nice and friendly and we haven't got to anything which is contentious.

This meant that the joint governance arrangements developed for STPs, such as system leadership groups, had remained largely untested as vehicles for joint decision-making during the course of our research. It also created what one leader described as 'a veneer of collaboration' – with organisations appearing to work well together while tensions remained hidden beneath the surface. Leaders were clear that difficult decisions would need to be taken in future, but were rarely clear on how this would be done in practice. Some leaders were sceptical that these decisions would be made without more directive action from STP leaders. As one STP leader told us: 'you can't do this by committee'. Another told us that 'you're going to have to put somebody in overall charge to start driving it'. Future leadership of STPs is discussed in more detail below.

In one area with a limited history of collaboration between organisations, an independent facilitator had been put in place to help leaders discuss some of these 'sticky issues' at their system leadership group meetings. This was seen as a useful way to help overcome tensions and begin to make progress on issues where agreement (or even discussion) had been difficult in the past. An independent facilitator had also been used to run workshops in another of our STP areas and, again, was seen to have made a positive impact in progressing discussions.

Policy and structural challenges

Existing NHS policy and legislation on accountability and performance management provided more fundamental challenges to leaders' ability to work together on STPs. Leaders talked about the tension between being asked to collaborate on STPs while still being held to account as individual organisations. This was described as the 'fourth gap' to be addressed by STPs by leaders in one area (the other three being gaps in care quality, health and wellbeing, and NHS finances, as described in the original planning guidance). By this they meant the gap between existing accountability arrangements in the NHS – where legitimacy and accountability sits with individual organisations – and the new kind of collective governance arrangements needed to implement service changes between organisations.

This tension was most clearly expressed in relation to the accountability of NHS providers, who face strong incentives to improve their organisation's own performance and only weak incentives to collaborate. As one leader commented:

> *How do you make [place X] as a whole become financially sustainable? Within that you probably don't care whether one provider is or isn't because you can do the deals within that to make sure it all works for the NHS. The accountability, though, I would say is still 95 to 99 per cent holding those individual organisations to make sure they hit their bottom line.*

Organisations had no clarity about how they would be collectively held to account for their performance through STPs:

> *The CQC's [Care Quality Commission] process is not based on system work, it's based on individual organisational working – as is NHS Improvement's performance frameworks. So when you try to encourage people to forget their organisational boundary and work across sectors in a more fluid way, the first question you get asked quite often is: but if something goes wrong, who's accountable? And at the moment we haven't got an answer for that question, because the governance framework for the NHS is not set up in that way.*

This challenge was also recognised by our interviewees from NHS England's regional teams, who described the barriers to joint working created by their own performance management frameworks:

On the one hand we are asking these systems to work… across systems. Then I, as NHS England, and my colleagues in NHSI [NHS Improvement], are holding the organisations to account to deliver today and not taking a system view of it.

The role of national NHS bodies in the STP process is explored in more detail in Section 7.

From all parts of the system, the authority of individual organisations was seen to take precedence over any system-wide governance arrangements developed for the STP. In practice, there seemed to be no real delegation of authority from individual organisations to system leadership groups. As one NHS provider leader told us: 'all of the acute provider boards aren't delegating responsibility to anybody'. This lack of authority hampered the ability of STP leaders to make progress on key decisions:

You know, being honest, it would be much easier if I could say to all the trusts and CCGs, 'I want you to do this and I want that piece of work done by X and I want you to go to that meeting and I want you to come to this meeting and by the way this is going to be the approach to this back-office service – we agree a plan, we implement it'. I've got no direct authority over anybody.

Without any formal authority to make decisions on behalf of the system, leaders recognised the importance of softer leadership styles, such as negotiation and persuasion, to try to gain agreement and consensus between organisations. This is explored in more detail below.

Future governance of STPs

These governance challenges are expected to become more severe as the STP process moves from planning, to agreement of service changes, and on to implementation. Leaders recognised that the governance processes they had developed to support their STPs so far had primarily been designed around the need to write and agree a high-level plan, rather than to put that plan into practice. In our second round of interviews, leaders in most areas were reviewing how their governance processes could be strengthened to allow more formal decision-making to happen at an STP level. Interviewees told us that this would require organisations to pool some of their sovereignty, but were generally unclear on how this could be done within existing accountability frameworks.

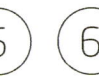   

A number of leaders called for action from national bodies to provide clarity on how these issues could be addressed in future. Questions were raised about whether organisational collaboration through STPs could be effective without more formal legislation underpinning it. For example, as one leader said:

> *If STPs are going to exist, are they going to continue as a collaboration, which are, by nature, actually optional, on one level (although all the money is going to be tied to the STP, so if you want any transformation money in the future you're going to have to be part of the STP, so it isn't optional either)? Or are you going to do something at a statute level, and create an entity called an STP?*

Some leaders felt that the creation of STP footprints already amounted to NHS restructuring – or, as one leader described it, 'legislation by the back door' – forcing organisations to collaborate across larger geographical areas. A number of leaders noted similarities between STPs and previous NHS structures such as regional health authorities and strategic health authorities (SHAs). Others recognised the 'mess' of current organisational arrangements in the NHS, but felt there was little appetite for more formal restructuring. STPs were therefore seen by some as a way to simplify these arrangements.

That said, some more formal organisational changes were already being discussed by NHS leaders as part of the STP process. In two areas, CCGs were actively exploring how they could work together to more formally commission services across their STP footprint. The form that these arrangements might take had not yet been agreed. Plans were also being developed by NHS providers to establish more formal governance arrangements between organisations, although these plans largely pre-dated the STP process. In one area, for example, NHS provider chief executives were exploring how they could establish a formal partnership between organisations delivering acute, community and mental health services.

The role of STP leaders

Leading the STP process has been challenging and time-consuming. Most STP leaders had found it difficult to manage their existing responsibilities alongside their STP leadership role – the exception being one leader who was already responsible for leading a major service transformation programme across the footprint before

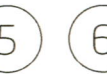   

STPs were announced. The time commitment for working on the STP has been significant. As one STP leader told us: 'I was supposed to be doing this one day a week. Actually I've been doing two full-time jobs in seven days.' Others said they were dedicating around three or four days a week to the role.

Achieving this balancing act between their day job and STP leadership has depended largely on the goodwill of leaders and additional support received from their colleagues. There was agreement, however, that this was unsustainable in the long term. As one leader told us, the job so far was 'not what I signed up for and it's not sustainable'. Practical support for leaders to carry out their role also seemed to be lacking: 'at the moment, they've set the STP up, said you're the lead, and that's it'. Some leaders and their boards were also concerned about the risks to their own organisation's performance as a result of time being spent on the STP:

> If they want to make a success of the STPs they've got to support the leaders and do it properly, and they can't expect us to do it on top of the day job because there will be no forgiveness if my trust goes down the pan because I'm concentrating on this. And, in fact, that's a discussion I've had with my board and executive directors have made the same point.

For their role to be manageable in future, STP leaders said they needed dedicated time and support – for example, by creating a full-time role for the STP leader, with an agreed set of responsibilities and teams to support them. They also talked about the need to be given more formal authority over local decision-making and powers to make changes to services in practice. The lack of authority of STP leaders was recognised as an issue by a range of interviewees from different organisations – not just the STP leaders themselves. For example, one interviewee said that:

> They haven't been appointed formally to that role, none of them, nor are they elected formally to that role, so there is a real governance issue beginning to bubble up.

STP leaders wanted clarity on these issues about their future role from national NHS bodies – but had not received it during the course of our research. This lack of clarity, combined with the pressures of doing the job, meant that some STP leaders were considering whether they would continue in the role in the future. As one said:

At some stage, certain people like me probably get to a position and say, 'actually, I am just going to go back to my day job', because it is quite a challenge doing all of this in a sea of fog.

For those working with them, the style and approach of STP leaders was important. Interviewees talked about the need for STP leaders to be collaborative, empathetic and able to engage a wide range of stakeholders in decisions, as well as being good communicators and influencers. At the same time, they also needed to be able to address difficult issues directly with their colleagues. Experience was important too – particularly in leading large-scale change and having an understanding of the whole health and care system. As one interviewee told us, this often requires a new set of skills from traditional NHS leaders:

So whereas, you know, the chief exec of one of the providers can just go and make it happen, actually, that's fine if it's in their organisation. But if it's not, then you have to do it through the negotiated approach. There really is different leaderships. We talk about different leadership needed [for] an integrated system – well, this is exactly the same sort of leadership that's needed.

Interviewees made the point that these behaviours needed to be developed by all leaders across the health and care system – not just the named STP leader. But while some chief executives were seen to be naturally collaborative in their approach, others needed to adapt their leadership style to be able to work more effectively across organisational boundaries.

Where leaders had a history of working together across the STP footprint, this provided a far stronger foundation for joint working on the STP and more collaborative and inclusive leadership styles. In one area in particular, leaders had worked together on a number of strategic initiatives in the past. The area had also experienced relative stability of senior leaders over a number of years. This meant that the task of building relationships and understanding the priorities of different leaders and organisations was far simpler compared with other STP areas. It also meant that leaders felt more able to cope with the inevitable tensions experienced throughout the STP process (*see* Section 5).

5 Who has been involved in developing STPs?

STP footprints cover many different organisations responsible for commissioning and providing services. Levels of involvement in the STP process between these organisations have varied – both between different parts of the health and care system and between STP areas. This section explores levels of involvement in the STP process at a local level from within the NHS, by local authorities, by patients and the public, and by other organisations. It also describes how leaders from these organisations worked together on STPs and some of the cultural and relational issues they faced in doing so, as well as the positive progress being made in building a sense of common purpose between leaders.

Involvement within the NHS

Despite STPs being an NHS planning initiative, levels of involvement and engagement in STPs by organisations from within the NHS have varied widely. Across all four STP areas involved in our research, the NHS organisations most actively involved in the STP process have been CCGs and major NHS providers (particularly acute providers). Leaders from these organisations have typically been involved in STP decision-making and governance processes, as well as being responsible for leading or contributing to work to develop the plans. The depth of involvement within these organisations, however, has typically been shallow, with clinical teams in particular often only weakly engaged in the process. This is explored in more detail below.

Within this picture, the involvement of NHS community and mental health service providers has been the most variable. In one of our STP areas, for example, a dedicated working group had been established to develop a mental health strategy for the STP area, involving a range of representatives from relevant services. In another area, however, mental health services had played a minimal role in the STP process so far – both in terms of the organisations involved and the focus of the

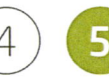
plans being developed. The involvement of these services depended heavily on local context and the history of collaboration within the footprint.

Across all four areas, those least involved in the process from within the NHS were GPs and primary care services. Leaders described how difficult it was to meaningfully engage general practice 'as a provider' in the process, given the large number of GPs in each area and the differences in views between them. The 'voice of primary care' was seen as a major gap in STP governance processes and work to develop the plans. For example, one interviewee described how primary care representatives were missing from key STP events:

> *If I were to look round and think about the people who were in the room at the stakeholder… the two stakeholder days, I couldn't say that there was anybody who I thought was representing primary care. So, I think they probably remain a hidden voice in all of this.*

Unsurprisingly, this meant that other issues tended to receive more attention:

> *I don't think we're talking enough about primary care. We're talking a lot about acute service configuration.*

Interviewees described the various routes they were using to try to engage GPs in the process. For some, CCG involvement was seen as a proxy for GP involvement. But most CCG leaders we interviewed were clear that they were involved in the STP process as commissioners rather than providers or primary care representatives. In areas where GP federations or large GP providers existed, they were seen as another route to access the views of primary care. But these groups were often 'emergent' forms of collaboration rather than well-established provider groups, and even where they did exist they were unable to speak on behalf of primary care across the whole STP footprint. At least two areas were also starting to try to engage GPs through local medical committees (LMCs).

Despite these efforts, none of our interviewees believed that their STP footprint had been successful in engaging primary care services in the plans so far. As one leader told us: 'It's so hard and so complex and we don't have the time.' Instead, some interviewees told us that GPs and primary care services needed to be engaged at a local level (for instance, in CCG areas) rather than through the STP programme.

Clinical engagement

As well as GPs and primary care teams, clinical engagement in STPs has also been weak. Clinical reference groups had usually formed part of STP governance structures, and various workshops had been held to try to involve clinicians at different points in the process. But most leaders told us that the tight timescales given to develop the plans had largely ruled out meaningful engagement with clinicians:

> *There is a number of meetings, but again… there is a real expectation that people just drop stuff for the STP meetings, when probably you won't get any clinical involvement. Because certainly consultants need six weeks' notice to be able to cancel a clinic, so the whole STP process is defaulted on that.*

Leaders also recognised the time it often takes for clinicians from different parts of the system to come together and build trust and relationships – particularly in areas with little history of collaboration between providers:

> *If you want to change community services, and pathways, and how hospitals work, you find the time for hospital consultants and GPs to go out for a meal, or do something informal and talk it through. Then, have some follow-up, formal, sort of, meetings… It will happen. But the whole… because, it's gone at such pace… I mean, everybody's assumed everybody knows each other, everybody assumes everybody knows how everybody else works.*

Leaders from all areas were concerned about the lack of clinical engagement in STPs so far. Securing deeper levels of engagement was a common priority, and interviewees recognised that 'nothing is going to happen' in practice if clinical teams are not actively involved in the process. At the same time, leaders also made the point that clinicians and frontline staff were already involved in various service improvement programmes within their footprint (for instance, at a CCG or trust level). Clinicians in two STP footprints, for example, had recently contributed to major clinical service reviews that were being used to inform the content of the STP. A lack of clinical involvement in the STP process directly, therefore, was not necessarily equated with a lack of clinical involvement in the content of the plans.

Involvement of local authorities

The strength and depth of local authority involvement in the plans has varied between STP footprints, ranging from strong involvement in decision-making and planning to very weak involvement in all aspects of the process.

In two of the four footprints involved in our research, local authorities have played a limited role in the process. While a small number of local authority leaders had attended STP meetings and been asked to provide comments on draft documents, they had typically played a minimal – and, in some cases, non-existent – role in developing the detail of the plans. Local authority leaders in these areas stressed that there is a difference between being informed about a plan (for instance, at a meeting) and being actively involved in developing it. They also described a range of issues with the way that NHS leaders had involved them in STP governance processes – for instance, by only involving one local authority leader in STP meetings and expecting them to speak on behalf of their colleagues from other areas. As one local authority chief executive told us: 'there's no way that talking to me gives you any mandate to decide how [another area] might be impacted by STP'.

When local government leaders in these areas were consulted on the STP, it was usually for particular elements of the plan rather than as equal partners in its overall development:

> *What seems to happen is that health recognises certain areas that are definitely local authority areas and they almost say: 'well, they are the areas that we're going to talk to you about'. Whereas actually, local authorities more and more have responsibility for the whole system, and so you need to be treated as an equal partner rather than a consultee on a section within the STP.*

As a result, local authority leaders in these two areas felt little ownership of the plan that was being developed. On the day of the draft STP submission in June, for example, one local authority chief executive told us: 'I mean, I don't even know what the STP looks like.'

This lack of involvement was a concern for local authority leaders. They recognised the impact that the plans could have on their local populations. They also highlighted the contribution that they could have made to the plans if they had been more involved in developing them. Some of their other colleagues, however, were far more dismissive of the STP process altogether. For example, one local government leader told us that:

> *The other [local authority] chief execs, they really just don't buy into this. The majority of chief execs in [place X] just think it's a joke.*

In our other two footprints, the involvement of local authorities in the STP process was far stronger. Unsurprisingly, the strongest level of local authority involvement was found in the STP footprint being led by a local authority leader. Interviewees from this area described high levels of collaboration between the NHS and local government, with one NHS leader describing the STP process as 'a refreshing, positive symmetry between local government and health'. While this was partly attributed to the good history of collaboration between the NHS and local government within the STP footprint, local authority leadership of the STP process was seen to be important too. Compared with other STP areas, the scope of the plan being developed in this area seemed to extend furthest outside the realms of the NHS – for example, with a dedicated working group focusing on housing and environmental issues.

Despite the wide variation in local authority involvement in STPs in practice, all NHS leaders talked about the importance of involving local authorities as much as possible in the process – even if this had not happened so far. The reasons offered were sometimes overtly political, with NHS leaders recognising the need to engage local politicians early when difficult decisions were likely to be made about acute hospital reconfigurations. The political dimension of the plans is explored in more detail in the box, p 41. The important role of local government in improving broader population health and wellbeing was also recognised by interviewees. NHS leaders also valued the experience of local government in managing significant budget cuts while maintaining services, as well as their skills in public engagement.

Where collaboration between the NHS and local government so far had been weak, a number of explanations were offered. For some interviewees, it was because relationships between the NHS and local government primarily existed at a local level (for example, between a single local authority and a CCG) rather than across the STP footprint. Replicating these local relationships across a wider geographical area was not always easy. For others, it was simply because the timescales to develop the plan were just too short to allow meaningful engagement – particularly given the pressures already facing local government. For example, local authority leaders told us that:

> *In delivering this to this timescale, I honestly don't see how they could have effectively engaged with the local politics of every local authority in the footprint area that they're servicing.*

> *They know that they need to involve local government, but they're so focused on the task of getting themselves sorted out so they can put in a submission, it's very difficult for them to do that.*

This means that the blame for a lack of engagement with local authorities often lay with national NHS bodies, rather than local leaders:

> *I don't blame the people on the ground up here for the fact that we don't feel engaged, I blame the pace that's being dictated by central government – the Department of Health somewhere I suspect.*

These criticisms did not stop at the STP timeline. Interviewees also told us that the national process had been 'exclusive of local authorities' – focusing primarily on NHS services and not considering the role that local authorities would play in developing the plans. The original STP planning guidance, for instance, contained only minimal references to local government and how they should be involved in the process. This meant that local government leaders were often unclear about the part they were expected to play in developing the plans.

Involvement of patients and the public

Patients and the public have been largely absent from the STP process so far. In all STP areas, leaders told us it was almost impossible to involve patients and the public effectively in the plans within the timescales available (or, as one leader told us, 'it's a complete no-hoper'). Patient and public involvement was therefore seen as something that local areas would need to do once their STPs had been submitted, rather than before.

We did find a small number of examples of patient representatives being involved in limited discussions about their local STP. This included members of Healthwatch attending meetings or STP steering groups, as well as patient and public representatives attending STP workshops. Some areas were also using local processes (such as patient and public involvement panels) to keep members of the public informed about the development of the plans. But despite these examples, leaders in all areas were clear that patient and public involvement in practice has been minimal. This was seen as a clear risk to the success of STPs. It also meant that the voice of 'real people' was missing from the process:

> *I've been in meetings where I've felt a little bit like, you know, where are the real people in this?*

As well as the timeline creating a barrier to meaningful public engagement, national NHS bodies had also asked STP leaders to keep details of draft STPs out of the public domain. This included instructions to actively reject Freedom of Information Act requests (FOIs) to see draft plans. Two main reasons were given for this. The first was that national NHS leaders wanted to be able to 'manage' the STP narrative at a national level – particularly where plans might involve politically sensitive changes to hospital services. The second was that national leaders did not want draft proposals to be made public until they had agreed on their content. Local leaders were typically unsupportive of this approach:

> *All the national guidance says don't share it, don't put in the public [domain] because people like [X national leader] and [X national leader] want to manage the national political messages to make sure that things like hospital closures and things like that don't get leaked... I think that's a bit of a wrong judgement call because I think at the end of the day, things will get leaked so it's better to actively involve people.*

> *One of the big risks is the ludicrous suggestion from the top that actually the documentation shouldn't be shared at this stage, it should be kept private and confidential.*

> *So there is potential, because of this hold on engagement, that they'll get it [their STP] all signed off, just about, and then they'll just have a massive fight.*

That said, in areas where major hospital reconfigurations were being planned, some NHS leaders did agree that details of specific changes should be kept private until formal public consultations could be launched. This was primarily for legal reasons. Leaders from some areas also thought that public involvement in STPs would create 'engagement fatigue', given the range of other initiatives planned or under way within local areas. As one leader told us: 'I struggle to get my head around this plethora of initiatives – and explaining that to the public – it's just… their eyes roll.' Others made the related point that various parts of their STP were based on pre-existing local plans, which had already been developed in collaboration with patients and the public. Notwithstanding these caveats, leaders in all areas were worried that the lack of meaningful public engagement in the plans would be damaging for the process.

Involvement of the voluntary sector and private providers

Engagement with the voluntary sector throughout the STP process has also been limited. Like with patients and the public, representatives from voluntary sector organisations had sometimes been involved in STP workshops and meetings. But they had rarely played a significant role in developing the detail of the plans.

The challenge of engagement between the NHS and the voluntary sector seemed to be two-way. Interviewees talked about the difficulties of knowing how to access and engage with a large number of disparate voluntary sector organisations across their area. Voluntary sector organisations also seemed to find it difficult to engage with the NHS. As one leader told us: 'they would want to be engaged, but they find it hard to find the right place and the right mechanisms for their voices to be heard'. For these reasons, voluntary sector engagement typically seemed to have been put on the 'too hard to do' pile, as one leader described it.

The exception to this rule was found in one STP footprint, where the leader of a social enterprise providing community services was responsible for leading the development of part of the draft STP. But even in this area, broader voluntary sector engagement (beyond organisations providing core NHS services) in the process had been weak.

The same was true for representatives from private sector providers. While some private providers were involved in STP workshops in areas where they already delivered services – for instance, out-of-hours providers – the involvement of private providers in the STP process was limited across our four areas. In most cases, this was simply because of the peripheral role that these providers played in their local system. The involvement of private sector management consultants, however, was much more widespread and is explored in Section 6.

Relationships and behaviours

Regardless of which organisations had been more or less involved in the process, all STP areas had experienced tensions between organisations and leaders when developing the plans. These tensions were typically seen as an inevitable consequence of organisations being asked to collaborate in a policy environment that was not designed to support joint working. The ability of leaders to overcome these tensions was highly dependent on the strength of the relationships between them and their history of collaboration prior to the STP.

Tensions between acute providers in the NHS were common – especially when options for reconfiguring acute services were being considered as part of the STP, creating perceived 'winners' and 'losers' between different providers within the footprint. The annual contracting round in the NHS also created considerable tensions between commissioners and providers – being variously described as 'bruising', 'dreadfully dysfunctional' and 'an enormous waste of time' by CCG and provider leaders. These transactional discussions created a weak foundation for joint working on STPs. As one CCG leader explained:

> We've just had a very bruising contract negotiation round with the acute hospital, so they are very, very bruised, and they are now saying 'what is the point of us doing transformation?' The relationships are incredibly low.

Each STP footprint also experienced their own set of locally specific conflicts and tensions – for example, resulting from longstanding competitive behaviours between particular leaders and organisations. These tensions were rarely amenable to quick fixes, requiring time and effort on behalf of leaders to manage as the process went on. Tensions were also created by the manner in which STP leaders and footprints were defined, as described in Section 3.

Overcoming these kinds of relational and behavioural issues was generally seen as the most challenging part of the STP process, as well as the most important. But the

tight timescales available to develop the plans meant that the technical components of the process – such as developing governance arrangements or calculating the size of financial deficits – had often received more attention than the need to build trust and relationships across the system. Leaders recognised that far more attention needs to be paid to these relational and behavioural components of change in future – particularly in areas with little history of collaboration between organisations and leaders.

Positive progress and a sense of 'common purpose'

Interviewees also talked about the positive progress they were making – albeit slow, in some cases, or from 'a long way back' – in building relationships and strengthening partnerships across their local system. Leaders in most areas felt they had made progress in building a sense of 'common purpose' as the STP process has gone on, as well as a general commitment to collaborate to improve services:

> *On the whole, people are trying to work together, and whilst there are some natural tensions, people are collectively trying to do the right thing.*

> *I think there is a sense of common purpose there and people are getting on and working together and to some extent overcoming some of those sort of historical things.*

Some leaders said that the STP process had been a useful catalyst for establishing a 'common purpose' and engaging different parts of their health and care system in local planning processes. In one of the four areas, where organisations were already used to working together across the STP footprint, the process had been seen as an important and welcome opportunity to accelerate existing plans for service changes and develop momentum behind these plans. The STP had also been used by NHS leaders in this area as a way to draw colleagues from local government into discussions about planning for the future.

Across all four STP areas, we found a general agreement among leaders that collaborating to improve services and manage limited resources was the right thing to do. This meant that, despite the range of issues with the STP process and the tensions experienced along the way, leaders were typically committed to working together to address common challenges.

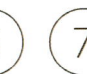

The political dimension of sustainability and transformation plans

Leaders from all STP areas recognised the potential political problems that their plans might face once they became public, at both a local and a national level.

At a local level, a number of NHS leaders were concerned about the potential reaction from the public and local politicians to the service changes being proposed in their STP. This was particularly true when STP footprints were considering reconfiguring acute hospital services – such as consolidating services currently provided on multiple sites, or downgrading accident and emergency (A&E) services. As one leader said, 'there is going to be noise' from local people and politicians when the plans are finalised and announced. The lack of extensive public engagement in the plans so far was seen to have added to this risk.

A small number of leaders also highlighted the potential political issues that would be created by STPs at a national level – again, particularly given the number of areas across the country making plans for reconfiguring acute hospital services. One leader said:

> So when we get to a point where we can clearly articulate the change, that's going to be a lot of quite difficult changes that are articulated all at the same time. Now, that's always been an issue, but that's now even more difficult given the fragility of the political system. So will there be appetite for political support, for example, to reduce the number of type one A&Es?

Interviewees hoped that national NHS leaders would provide political support for the changes being proposed in their area – or 'air cover', as some leaders described it – including by communicating the benefits of the potential changes to national politicians. The uncertainty created by the referendum result to leave the European Union, as well as the arrival of a new Prime Minister, led some leaders to question whether there would be political appetite for these changes. As one leader told us:

> And I still wondered, you know, before all of this, how much bottle they had and how much political knowledge they would withstand at any one time. Because, you know, it's going to be difficult in particular constituencies where change is required. But now, I think there's no possibility of doing any of that until the political leadership at a national level is settled.

6 How has the STP process been managed by local areas?

Significant amounts of time and energy have gone into managing the STP process at a local level. STPs are being developed alongside various other planning processes and strategic initiatives, as well as the day-to-day work of commissioning and providing health services. Making all of these things happen at the same time has been challenging – and sometimes impossible – relying in large part on the goodwill of staff and their intrinsic motivation to improve services. In this section we describe how the STP process was resourced and managed at a local level, as well as how teams worked together to set priorities for their plan.

People and resources

The STP areas involved in our research had not received any additional money from national NHS bodies to fund the development of their plans. This meant that local leaders needed to rely on existing staff and resources to manage the STP process. They typically did this by:

- creating new teams made up of staff from existing planning roles

- funding new roles for the STP process – for example, STP programme directors

- asking staff to do work on the STP on top of their existing responsibilities

- hiring management consultants and other external advisers.

The resources being invested to do this were often substantial. In one area, a team of 12 NHS staff had been put in place to lead the STP programme management office, supplemented by a number of working groups involving staff from different parts of the system. In another area, at least £500,000 had been invested to manage

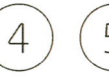
the STP process up to July 2016; leaders estimated that this would need to grow to around £3 million to manage it over the following year. In most cases, these arrangements had taken time to put in place – sometimes needing funding to be agreed between different organisations – and meant resources being diverted away from other initiatives or local priorities. Even in one area where formal programme management arrangements had not been put in place, leaders and their teams were still investing a significant proportion of their time to work on the STP.

Despite this, most leaders still felt that they did not have the resources they needed to develop a sufficiently detailed plan. Teams were having to juggle work on the STP with other full-time responsibilities, relying heavily on the goodwill of staff to manage the additional workload. One leader told us that: 'given the scale of this programme, it's nowhere near sufficiently resourced'. The scale of investment required was also expected to grow as the process moved from planning to implementation.

Management consultants

Management consultants were being used to support the development of STPs in three out of our four areas. The reasons for this varied. Sometimes they were used to fill gaps in NHS capacity – for example, where there were not enough NHS staff available at short notice to work on the STP. In other cases, they were used to fill perceived gaps in NHS capability – for example, providing specialist expertise in financial modelling. Some areas were using more than one management consulting firm for different parts of the STP, as well as receiving support from commissioning support units (CSUs) and academic health science networks (AHSNs). Even in the one STP area that had not directly commissioned external support to develop its plan, NHS England's regional team had commissioned a management consulting firm to carry out analytical work on behalf of its STP areas. The use of external advisers to support the planning process was routine.

Some leaders felt that STPs had 'created an industry' for management consultants – and questions were raised about why money is being invested in advice from private companies instead of in frontline services. In one area, STP leaders even felt under pressure from NHS England's regional team to increase the amount of money they were spending on management consultancy support. One leader told us they were 'picked out' for not spending enough on their STP programme, compared with other STP areas in the region.

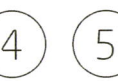

Leaders questioned whether this kind of reliance on management consultants was sustainable in future. As well as expressing concerns about the financial implications of continuing to use management consultants, leaders recognised the need for STP areas to build their own capacity and capability to support the implementation of their plans.

Responding to the national process

The day-to-day management of the STP process by local teams largely centred on the need to meet various national planning deadlines. Draft documents needed to be produced, discussed at meetings or workshops, and circulated to key individuals before they could be submitted to regional or national NHS bodies. The timelines for doing this were tight – and, for most leaders, unrealistic. Multiple draft plans were being produced in quick succession to respond to local and national feedback; leaders from one area talked about producing around five draft plans a week ahead of the June planning deadline – sometimes being circulated in the early hours of the morning. In this context, getting meaningful engagement on the content of plans from a variety of people was difficult – often being done by email and at the last minute:

> It's not enough to say 'that's what's going in tomorrow'. That's not involvement, that's not engagement with the process. That's just us doing something and then just sharing it at the last minute. But that's the timeframe.

> I'd probably say, by definition, you should never manage by email, and I'd say the whole STP has been managed by email... And it's cheap management – 'if you don't come back to us by this time or date then it's taken as it's agreed'. I mean, every timeline is just silly, it's normally one and a half/two days' turnaround.

As well as the tight timelines creating difficulties for local teams, interviewees also described the challenges created by the way that the process was managed by national NHS bodies. Planning guidance and templates often arrived late. Expectations for the plans seemed to change and grow over time. And the process for submitting and redrafting plans was often unclear and subject to change. These issues made local management of the process more difficult, and are described in more detail in Section 7. Some areas were better able to cope with these challenges than others. In one STP footprint, well-established programme management arrangements already existed to lead system-wide changes to services. This eased the process of managing the day-to-day work on the STP.

A number of interviewees commented on the large proportion of their time that seemed to be spent responding to requests from national NHS bodies rather than focusing on the detail of developing their plans. STP areas were asked to complete and submit various draft plans and templates throughout the STP process. This consumed staff time and effort. As one leader said: 'the risk is that you start to manage a process rather than develop a meaningful plan'. Another leader – echoing the comments of others from different footprints – thought that time and energy was being wasted 'feeding the beast':

> *But it's so much of our time and energy with these f***ing documents… feeding the beast when it's the beast that feeds you through NHS Improvement, NHS England. I mean, the time my staff spend on creating documentation is just grim.*

Managing existing work alongside the STP

Leaders and staff in all areas struggled to manage their existing workloads and priorities alongside work on the STP. For some organisations – particularly NHS providers – managing current financial and service pressures while also being involved in the STP has been a big challenge in itself. This was particularly true in areas where NHS providers were under pressure from regulators to improve performance and meet organisational targets. Interviewees from local government also told us about the difficulties of finding time to work on STPs when they face significant pressures of their own.

For many organisations, STPs were also being developed alongside a number of other transformation initiatives, such as vanguard sites, devolution plans, organisational mergers, and other local integration programmes. This was true in all four of our STP areas. It meant that leaders and staff had to balance their time between multiple initiatives and plans, often on top of their day-to-day work. Making this balancing act work in practice was not always possible, and often meant prioritising the STP over other initiatives. For example, one CCG leader described how work on their local integration programme – which had been in development for nearly two years – had been put on hold so that staff could work on the STP:

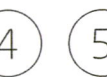

It's stopped, yes, it's literally stopped. And both in terms of people's time, energy, it's just stopped.

A lack of clarity about the relationship between various programmes and initiatives made this balancing act more difficult to achieve. This lack of clarity was partly caused by differences in boundaries and timelines between initiatives – for example, devolution plans were often being developed across different areas to STPs, as well as to different deadlines. But it was also caused by local leaders not knowing which initiatives took precedence in the eyes of national NHS leaders. For example, should leaders prioritise work on existing vanguard programmes, or should they instead be working on the STP? And what about plans for devolution? While leaders recognised the links between these programmes, they often talked about the choices that needed to be taken about where to focus their limited time and energy.

Leaders in some areas were also concerned that future funding for their local transformation work would now be reliant on STPs. In one area, for example, leaders from local government were told by NHS England that funding for their devolution plan was now conditional on developing an acceptable STP across a wider geographical footprint. This caused some frustration within local government – particularly given that these devolution plans pre-dated work on STPs. Similar tensions existed for some vanguard programmes.

Setting priorities and developing the plan

The process of setting priorities for STPs varied across our four footprints. Some areas started by understanding the 'gaps' in health care quality, health outcomes and finances in their area, and used these to identify priority areas for their STP. A number of leaders commented that closing gaps in NHS finances seemed to be the key priority for national NHS bodies, particularly as the process went on (*see* Section 7). Other footprints primarily used existing plans or initiatives – both across the footprint and in local areas – as the foundation for their STP, rather than identifying 'new' priorities *per se*. This was particularly the case where plans for service changes already existed across the STP footprint – as in one of our areas in particular – making the local planning and decision-making process far simpler than in other areas. In reality, each footprint used a combination of approaches to set their STP priorities, but the balance between 'old' and 'new' priorities varied between areas.

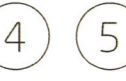
For most leaders, the process of planning across multiple organisations and areas has not been simple. Two footprints in particular have struggled to make their STP more than just a sum of pre-existing local plans. Some leaders saw planning at an STP level as 'a game' to be played to secure transformation funding to be able to carry on with their own local initiatives. Others were more positive about the opportunity to join together different local plans and identify common elements for improvement between them.

Whichever way priorities were established, reconfigurations of acute hospital services (of different varieties) were often high up the agenda. This was not always welcome. Many leaders were concerned that not enough attention was being paid to primary and community services and the wider determinants of health. Leaders from various parts of the health and care system talked about the imbalance in their plans towards acute hospital services. There was a sense among some leaders that broader priorities were often getting lost in a drive to achieve financial balance and in the context of growing pressures on acute services:

> *Actually it feels to me as though we've got to turn the whole thing on its head and to think much more around actually what are we going to do to actually invest in community and build resilience, really up the prevention agenda, think about how we redesign health and social care together, building up primary care, community care. That feels to me as though it's getting lost in this drive for: 'you've got to make it balance and the only way you can do that is through the acute reconfiguration'.*

> *We are a system, like a lot of them, where it feels as though the pressure will keep reverting, will keep reverting to urgent care, and that I'm going to have to keep pushing and saying, 'let's keep it much broader'.*

When draft STPs were produced, leaders in all areas commented that their plans were 'high level' and lacking in detail on how broad principles (such as strengthening primary and community services) would be put into practice. This was seen as an inevitable consequence of the timescales that had been given to develop the plan – as well as the need to keep key details of service changes (where they existed) out of the public domain. But it meant that leaders often only felt ownership of the broad vision or 'case for change' set out in the STP, rather than any specific service changes to be implemented. For example, one leader said:

What there isn't is any granular plan. What there isn't is any substance that will show how it's to be done. Who can argue with maximising prevention, sort of, getting into health promotion and treating people closer to home and all the rest of it? Everybody agrees with that but it's what you mean by it and how you make it happen, and that's what's missing.

More detail, however, was required of local leaders when submitting financial templates to national NHS bodies. Each STP footprint had been asked to complete a spreadsheet setting out how they would achieve financial balance in future. These spreadsheets focused on NHS finances rather than combined gaps in NHS and local government finances, which was an issue for some local leaders who had wanted to take a broader approach to local finances. These templates were not submitted by all four of our STP areas in time for the initial deadline (June 2016). But for those areas that did, many local leaders did not feel confident about the assumptions and analysis underpinning their projections. Again, leaders told us that developing credible projections for system-wide finances in the time available was difficult. As one NHS provider sector leader said:

So, if you think about all that productivity and such like, over a longer time period, you could probably have facilitated it, and done a really good OD [organisational development]/development piece with the respective finance directors in [footprint X]. They never get the chance to meet together. If they got to a stage of, 'let's actually do open book with each other, and then talk it through properly', you could make real credible progress about how the financial sustainability comes together. But within that timeframe, you've either got, at best, deputy finance directors in the room, or associate finance directors, who probably had five minutes in a corridor with their finance director… and that's the same for every piece, whether it be workforce, or any of these things, or estates… If you're going to do it you might as well do it well, and if you're going [to] do it well, you can never do it in two months, or whatever we've tried to do it in.

The challenge recognised by leaders in all areas was how to turn their high-level STP drafts into more detailed plans that could be implemented in 2017. Local leaders were hoping that this detail could be developed in time for their final plan to be submitted in October 2016, but recognised that even the final plan was likely to need further work and consultation.

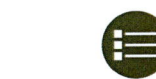

How has the process been managed by national NHS bodies?

National NHS bodies have been responsible for the overall direction and management of STPs across England. While local leaders were generally supportive of the broad idea behind the STP process, they experienced a number of issues with the way it has been led and managed at a national level. In this section we describe local leaders' perceptions of the overall management of the STP process, the fragmentation often experienced in the approaches taken by national NHS bodies, and the role played by national bodies in establishing priorities for the plans.

Process and guidelines

Interviewees were generally critical of the way the STP process had been managed by NHS England and other national bodies. Guidance promised to support areas to develop their plans typically arrived late and, in some cases, never materialised at all. When guidance or templates were produced, local leaders told us that they often created ambiguity over what the plans should include. For example, STP guidance simultaneously asked leaders to address a long list of national requirements while also focusing on a small number of priority areas. The guidance also often arrived too late for leaders and their teams to adequately respond within the allotted timescale. Detailed financial templates, for instance, arrived at the beginning of June – less than a month before they were due to be submitted.

The timelines and expectations for the plans also changed over time. Planning deadlines were revised as the process went on, and leaders typically had very little knowledge of how future stages of the process – for example, assessment of their plans – would work in practice. The list of requirements for what should be covered in STPs has also grown. At the end of June 2016, for instance – just days before draft plans were due to be submitted to national bodies – letters were issued by NHS Improvement calling on STP leaders to include plans for consolidating back-office and pathology services in their STPs. This created a sense for some leaders that the scope of STPs was continually growing; as one leader described it: 'every issue, every problem, everything that is raised will be sorted out through the STP'. It also meant that the focus of local leaders was constantly being pulled in different directions:

> *Monday we're told we're straight, on Wednesday it's turn right, Friday it's do a U-turn.*

Even when deadlines were changed to give leaders more time to produce a final plan, most felt that the timelines given to complete their STPs have been unrealistic. Leaders were concerned about their ability to develop a meaningful plan within the timescales available. They were also concerned about the amount of time spent 'managing the process' rather than the detail of the plan (*see* Section 6). While leaders recognised the need for pace in meeting the challenges facing local services – and, in some cases, said that speed of the process had galvanised local partnerships – we were told that there needs to be a balance between 'pace and reality'. The tight timescales in which to develop the plans caused a variety of problems for local leaders – for example, in securing widespread involvement in the process (*see* Section 5).

This combination of issues gave many local leaders the impression that NHS England and other national bodies lacked a clear plan for STPs. One leader said that national bodies seemed to be 'making it up as they go'. Another said: 'sometimes it just doesn't feel like they know what they are doing'. One leader described the process as 'a shambles'. More importantly, interviewees felt that the way the process was being managed at a national level was making the task of developing STPs more difficult. One leader told us that 'effectively we're trying to do a good job in spite of the centre's approach rather than because of it'.

These negative attitudes towards the management of the process contrasted with the more positive attitudes of local leaders towards the principle of STPs. Interviewees were typically supportive of the concept of working together to develop plans for the future, and recognised the need to collaborate to meet the challenges facing local services:

> *So I think inherently the concept is a good one – (a) of the STP and (b) of… balancing service considerations with citizen outcomes and money, broadly. That's*

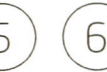

the fairly decent thing to do, as well as taking a run at these things and trying to have a longer-term plan and view of it. So I think that's good.

They simply felt the process had been poorly managed – or, as one leader said, 'the right thing being done badly'. At the same time, local leaders also recognised the difficult context in which national NHS leaders were operating – both in terms of the slowdown in growth of NHS funding and growing pressure from the Department of Health and the Treasury to bring the NHS back into financial balance.

Regional support and co-ordination with national teams

Issues with the national management of the process were compounded by a lack of alignment between NHS England's national and regional teams in supporting STP areas. In one area, for example, NHS England's regional team had produced their own guidance for STP leaders, setting out expectations for what should be included in the plans. Subsequent national guidance contradicted these instructions, creating conflicting requirements and additional work for STP leaders.

Examples like these were also highlighted by interviewees from NHS England, who in some regions felt actively excluded from the STP process and 'bypassed' by national teams. This in turn made their job of supporting STP leaders more difficult, as they often lacked the right information about what was being asked of local leaders and how the plans would be assessed. This fragmentation seems to have been most acute at the start of the process, with some leaders reporting an improvement in co-ordination during our second round of interviews.

The approach taken by NHS England's regional teams in supporting the STP process varied across the country. Some regional teams sought to exert far more control over the process and the content of the plans than others. In one STP area in particular, leaders told us that the regional team's approach felt interventionist and 'top-down'. The regional team had asked STP leaders to complete various documents and templates in addition to the national process, often within unrealistic timescales: 'there is a tendency to fall into the whole, you know, "we need a 10-page slide pack by tomorrow"'. This left some leaders feeling disempowered by the process.

In other areas, interviewees were more positive about the supportive role that NHS England regional teams have played at different points throughout the process. This included being involved in STP leadership meetings, reviewing draft plans, and helping local leaders prepare for their STP review meetings with national leaders. Regional teams had also organised various events to try to share learning between different STP footprints and secure deeper engagement in the process. While NHS Improvement's regional teams had begun to play a greater role in the process as it went on (for example, attending STP meetings), and were working with NHS England's regional teams to do this, NHS England seemed to be playing the leading role in providing regional support for the STP process. It is worth recognising that NHS Improvement as an organisation was in a process of transition throughout our research.

Tensions between NHS Improvement and NHS England

Interviewees described tensions in the approaches taken between NHS England and NHS Improvement throughout the STP process, and the impact this was having on their ability to work together. As described in Section 4, local leaders talked about the governance challenges of being asked to work collectively on STPs while still being held to account as individual organisations. Unsurprisingly, this tension was being played out in practice in our STP areas – with NHS Improvement often being seen to prioritise improvements in NHS provider performance over system-wide performance through STPs. CCG leaders in particular felt that 'unhelpful' conversations were taking place between NHS Improvement and NHS providers – particularly in relation to the need to reduce financial deficits.

For STPs to work in practice, interviewees talked about the changes needed in how national NHS bodies work together to support collaboration between organisations, rather than reinforcing the barriers between them. For example, one interviewee from NHS England said:

> *This is another part of the governance picture – not just how they [local NHS organisations] arrange themselves to be able to do this in collaboration, but actually how we, as regulators, arrange ourselves around them, so that we don't undermine it.*

Some interviewees felt that alignment was stronger at the top of NHS England and NHS Improvement – for example, between Jim Mackey, Chief Executive of NHS Improvement, and Simon Stevens, Chief Executive of NHS England. Both of these

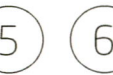

leaders had attended meetings with STP leaders at different points in the process to discuss draft plans and key issues to be addressed (*see* Appendix). But this alignment was not always mirrored within their organisations and in the approaches taken in practice to regulation and performance management of different parts of the NHS.

The priorities of national bodies

While guidance produced by national NHS bodies had provided long lists of priorities for local areas to address in their STPs, many interviewees felt that the top priority for national leaders was increasingly 'the money' – and, in some cases, 'acute trust reconfiguration and the money'. Midway through the STP process, leaders had been asked to complete detailed financial templates setting out how their plans would close gaps in local NHS finances. Feedback on draft plans from national bodies also often focused on how the changes being proposed would deliver financial savings – in some cases encouraging NHS leaders to be more ambitious in thinking about what could be achieved.

Leaders in one area, for instance, were asked to revisit their initial plans because they had not been able to show how they would close the significant gap in local NHS finances:

> But the reason really to go back and revisit a lot of this was, to be frank, on the basis of the feedback from the [X national leader] discussion which was, you know, 'your staff have to deliver the £[X] million gap and anything that doesn't answer that question really isn't going to cut it'.

The scale of the financial savings required often meant that local leaders were exploring changes to acute services as a major part of their STP, alongside other organisationally based programmes (such as provider cost-improvement programmes) to improve efficiency. One interviewee described how there seemed to be two narratives about the STP process from national NHS bodies: the formal narrative set out in the planning guidance, focused on a wide range of services and priorities; and the informal 'messages' to local areas, focused on saving money and making changes to acute hospital services. These informal messages had a clear impact on the content of the plans being produced by local leaders.

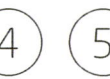

8 How will local areas make change happen?

Across all STP areas, leaders were concerned about their ability to turn the vision being articulated in their STP into reality. Interviewees described how the process so far had been fundamentally geared towards producing a plan, with little time to think in detail about how the objectives in the plan would be met. For some leaders, this worryingly echoed the experience of previous planning initiatives in the NHS, where bold visions had been created but implementation had been weak. As one leader said:

> *We've got a really, really good history of producing the most fantastic glossy award-winning plans… The weak bit is the implementation bit. And that's the bit I'm worried about. The big focus is on 'getting the plan, getting the plan, getting the plan', and I'm thinking, 'I'm not bothered about the plan; I'm bothered about the moving to implementation', and that's the scary bit.*

Leaders questioned whether they had the right skills and resources available at a local level to implement their plans. Interviewees described the upfront investment required to implement key parts of their plan, both in terms of capital investment and money to fund the double-running of services while new models of care are developed. They also talked about the need to release staff from their day-to-day work to design and implement improvements to services – particularly clinicians and other frontline staff. Dedicated programme management resources would also be needed to oversee the delivery of the plans. As one leader said: 'The main challenge is going to be how to do this alongside doing the day job. It's just terrifying.' Some leaders were also concerned about whether they had people with the right skills within their system to manage and co-ordinate complex service changes.

These concerns about weak implementation of the plans were also linked to the lack of engagement in STPs so far (*see* Section 5), the need to build relationships between leaders, and the potential political problems caused by STPs (*see* box, p 41). There

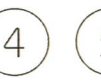

was a sense among many leaders that, despite the challenges they had experienced in managing the STP process so far, the real challenges were yet to come. As one leader said:

> *It's really easy agreeing in principle. It's really easy in terms of direction of travel. I mean, there is nothing new in what's been said in [place X] in terms of the STP […] that isn't in the five year Forward View or any number of other publications, but it's when you actually bring it down to, well, this means choices. This means decisions. This means choice of where you actually spend or don't spend. It means curtailing of some services in order to actually develop others. That's where it… or decisions between organisational interests, that's where the difficulty is. We haven't got to those points.*

These questions will be explored in more detail in the second phase of our research.

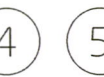
9 Discussion

STPs are based on the idea that collective action is needed to address the significant pressures facing health and care services in England. As we have argued elsewhere: this logic is good (Alderwick and Ham 2016; Ham and Alderwick 2015). New models of care are needed that span organisational boundaries within the NHS and between the NHS and local government. Improving population health and wellbeing requires co-ordinated action across the public sector and beyond. And doing both of these requires organisations to collaborate to make the best use of the limited resources available for improving health and care services.

The findings of this report highlight some of the difficulties experienced in making these ideas work in practice in the NHS today. While local NHS leaders are supportive of the idea of working together to improve care and manage limited resources, they have been highly critical of the way the STP process has been managed at a national level. Expectations and timelines for the plans have changed over time, guidance has often arrived late, and there have been inconsistencies in the approaches taken by different national NHS bodies.

These issues have made the already difficult task of developing STPs even more challenging. STP leaders and local teams have invested significant amounts of time and energy into developing their plans, often on top of their day jobs and other local initiatives. Making the STP process work has relied in large part on the goodwill and intrinsic motivation of staff – although some leaders wonder how long this will last without additional resources to ease the pressure on their local teams. Most areas have made progress in developing relationships and a sense of 'common purpose' among leaders within the footprint, with the STP being seen as a useful catalyst for achieving this. The importance of this should not be understated. But deeper engagement in the process is needed and the detail behind draft plans is often lacking.

While many of our findings are critical of the STP process and its evolution, they need to be set in context. Given the significant financial and service pressures facing NHS and social care services, the fact that leaders have made any progress on their

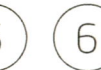

plans is an achievement in itself – particularly given the tight timescales involved. STPs are also being developed in an NHS environment that was not designed to support collaboration between organisations. In many ways, STPs represent a complex 'workaround' to the fragmentation and complexity introduced by the Health and Social Care Act. In this context, significant credit needs to be given to NHS and local government leaders involved in STPs for what has been achieved so far; it is no exaggeration to say that STPs could have failed to get out of the starting blocks without the hard work and commitment of local leaders.

It is also important to recognise the challenges faced by national NHS leaders throughout the STP process. As well as working within the constraints of the Health and Social Care Act, they are under pressure from central government to close gaps in NHS finances – at a time when the NHS faces an unprecedented slowdown in funding and dramatic cuts have been made to public health and social care budgets.

Unsurprisingly, local context and the history of collaboration within STP footprints have also played a major role in determining the progress of the plans. Where good relationships already existed between organisations – for instance, between the NHS and local government – these provided a foundation for positive collaboration on the STP. Some areas were also able to take forward and build on pre-existing plans for service changes in their STP. Where relationships across the STP footprint were poor, securing engagement in the process has been a major challenge in itself. This means that draft STPs are at widely different stages of development. Looking ahead, it also means that national NHS bodies will need to consider the different types of support needed for STP footprints after their final plans are submitted. Leaders from all four areas are concerned about their ability to implement the plans.

This report has painted a detailed picture of how the STP process has been managed and led up to July 2016 in four parts of the country. As well as helping us understand how local plans have been developed, our findings also provide important lessons for the future of STPs and raise questions about the broader policy environment in which they are being developed. These are explored below, along with recommendations about what needs to be done to improve the STP process.

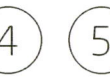   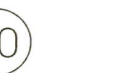
Strengthen involvement in the process

A clear conclusion from our research is that much broader and deeper engagement in STPs is needed in future. Within the NHS, clinicians and other frontline staff in particular need to be actively involved in developing plans for improving services. Previous experience in the NHS (Wilkinson *et al* 2011) suggests this will not be a simple task. But ambitious goals for improving quality of care described in STPs are unlikely to be met without deeper involvement of the people responsible for delivering those services.

The involvement of local authorities in developing STPs has varied significantly between areas. This should be a concern for national and local leaders. If STPs are to improve the health and wellbeing of their local populations, local authorities will need to be seen as core partners in developing and implementing the plans. At a local level, this will require NHS and local government leaders to decide how joint governance arrangements can be developed that properly take into account the voice of local government and the differences in accountability between the two systems. In areas with little history of joint working, it will also require time to build relationships and a shared understanding of how the NHS and local government can work together to achieve common goals. National NHS bodies will also need to pay far more attention to the role of local government in their overall management of the STP process – for instance, in STP guidance and timelines.

One of our interviewees recalled being in STP meetings and asking themselves: 'where are the real people in this?' The same question could be asked for the STP process as a whole. The answer, unfortunately, based on our research, is that patients and the public have been largely absent from the planning process so far. There appear to be two main reasons for this: a lack of time for adequate engagement, and instructions from national NHS bodies to keep details of draft plans out of the public domain. Whatever the reasons, a key priority now needs to be for local leaders to involve 'real people' in the development of their STP. Without this, the 'avoidable ignorance' about people's preferences so often experienced at the front lines of care (Mulley *et al* 2012) will be replicated across 44 STPs. Albeit late in the process, NHS England has now called on STP areas to involve the public in their plans (NHS England *et al* 2016). A range of approaches exists to support local leaders to do this (Coulter 2010; Foot *et al* 2014).

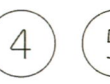

Strengthen STP governance and leadership

For STPs to work in practice, NHS organisations and their partners will need to find ways to make collective decisions about the use of resources and how services should be delivered. But doing this is not simple. As we described above, the major challenge in doing this is that STPs are being developed in an environment that was not designed to support collaboration between organisations. NHS organisations are held to account for individual rather than collective performance. Formal decision-making powers sit with these individual organisations rather than new STP footprints. And local authorities have altogether separate accountability arrangements to the NHS, including through the democratic accountability of elected councillors. There is therefore a major gap between existing accountability arrangements in the NHS and the kind of collective governance arrangements needed for STPs to function.

Our research has shown that this gap is not just theoretical. STP areas are finding it difficult to make decisions between multiple organisations, and no real delegation of responsibility from individual organisations to system leadership groups seems to be taking place in practice. While STP leaders have been appointed to oversee the development of their local plan, they have no real authority to make decisions on behalf of their system. In this context, interviewees told us that more formal governance arrangements were needed to support their STP in future – both to agree major service changes between organisations and to co-ordinate action to make them happen in practice.

But how will this be done? One argument could be made that developing collective governance arrangements for STPs should be left up to local areas themselves. This would allow arrangements to be developed to suit local context, and fits with evidence suggesting that locally developed rules and institutions play an important part in solving complex collective action problems (Ostrom 2010; Ostrom 1990). But this argument fails to recognise that many of the barriers to collaboration within the NHS lie outside the control of local leaders – resulting instead from national policies on accountability and performance management.

An alternative argument could be made that changes are needed in the way the NHS is structured to create more formal responsibilities for the leadership and management of NHS services across STP footprints. This would be one way to fill the vacuum in system leadership for NHS services left by the Health and Social Care Act, as well as providing clarity about the roles and responsibilities of STP footprints. But this argument is undermined by the previous experience of top-down structural reforms in the NHS, which have proved a major distraction from the task of improving frontline services (Ham *et al* 2015; Ham 2014).

For the time being, the right answer is likely to be found somewhere between these two extremes. While local organisations will need to agree on how they work together to achieve their aims (for example, agreeing a set of 'design principles' for improving services), national NHS bodies also need to play their part in removing the barriers that get in the way of local collaboration as STPs and new care models develop. For example, this means placing much more emphasis on holding systems to account for collective performance as well as holding organisations to account for individual performance. Changes to the statutory framework for the NHS may also be needed if STPs are going to be undermined by existing rules on competition and procurement – although there may be little appetite to do so.

National bodies also need to help STP areas understand the options available for collective decision-making and the role that NHS organisations should play in emerging systems of care. This might involve learning lessons from the experience of combined authorities in local government (Sandford 2016), as well sharing emerging lessons from areas like Greater Manchester and 'success regime' areas where thinking on these issues is most advanced. Lessons should also be learnt from the chequered experience of partnership arrangements in the public sector in the past (Audit Commission 2005).

The role of STP leaders within these new partnership arrangements also needs to be clarified and strengthened, particularly given our findings about the challenges experienced by those carrying out this role so far. This might include appointing full-time STP leaders – as is already happening in some areas through appointments or secondments – and establishing dedicated teams with sufficient resources to help them co-ordinate improvements in care between organisations. At the same time, leadership will need to be both shared and distributed across STP footprints for these improvements to be delivered in practice – recognising that making change happen in complex systems relies on alliances and collaborations rather than the actions of single heroic leaders (Timmins 2015; Senge *et al* 2015).

Provide co-ordinated national leadership

As well as developing local system leadership for STPs, there is also a clear need for closer alignment between national bodies in the NHS. In particular, our research has highlighted fragmentation between the approaches of NHS England and NHS Improvement in supporting local organisations and systems – for example, with NHS Improvement being seen to prioritise improvements in individual provider performance over system-wide performance. The recent single oversight framework produced by NHS Improvement (2016c) goes some way in shifting the balance of the NHS provider regulation towards STPs and systems of care, but the detail of the approach set out in the framework still focuses predominantly on how individual providers will be held to account for improving their own performance.

We have argued elsewhere that national NHS bodies should commit to producing their own '45th STP' – setting out how they will work together to provide a consistent and clear approach to supporting improvements in local areas (Ham 2016). Our research suggests that this would be far from tokenistic – and, indeed, would be welcomed by STP footprints. This might mean strengthening the role of the team established within NHS England to lead and co-ordinate work on the STP between different national bodies in the NHS. Better co-ordination is also needed between national and regional teams within NHS England.

Do not let short-term financial objectives crowd out work on new care models

The original purpose of STPs was to support local areas to implement the aims of the Forward View, including prioritising prevention and developing new models of integrated care. While these aims remain important to local leaders, the emphasis from national NHS bodies seems to have shifted over time to focus primarily on how STPs can bring the NHS into financial balance (quickly). This shift has been apparent throughout the course of our research, with STP leaders under pressure to show how their plans will close gaps in local finances. Analysis of draft plans also suggests that addressing financial deficits is an overriding priority for STP areas (Incisive Health 2016). Many are exploring reorganisations of acute hospital services to try to reduce costs, alongside other methods to try to improve efficiency – like standardising services, reducing unwarranted variations in care, and implementing other cost improvement programmes (Incisive Health 2016; Edwards 2016).

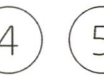
While closing gaps in NHS finances is undoubtedly important, there is a risk that plans for developing new models of care and prioritising prevention – things that are unlikely to deliver financial savings in the short term – will take a back seat. The added risk is that STPs will become dominated by bitter public debate about reconfigurations to acute hospital services, despite evidence suggesting that major reconfigurations of acute services rarely save money and sometimes fail to improve quality too (Imison *et al* 2014). If this happens, national leaders in the NHS will in turn find it difficult to explain to politicians why plans intended to accelerate integration of services and new models of care are now being used to support a different set of objectives that played little part in the Forward View.

Instead, STPs should be used as an opportunity to support and spread the new models of care already being developed by vanguards and other organisations right across the country. Areas such as Northumberland, Whitstable, Salford and Birmingham are developing new ways of delivering NHS and social care services to better meet the needs of their local populations (Collins 2016). But as our research has shown, maintaining work on these existing initiatives while also developing STPs has been difficult. National NHS bodies must provide clarity to local leaders that vanguards and other local initiatives remain an important part of the STP process. Leaders in these areas also need to be given time to show the benefits of the new models of care they are developing – and not held to account simply for short-term performance. The time needed to implement large-scale change in the NHS and to demonstrate its impact is often dramatically underestimated (Bardsley *et al* 2013; Steventon *et al* 2011).

Investment is also required to support these new models of care to develop and spread (Health Foundation and The King's Fund 2015). Yet additional funding for the NHS made available through the Sustainability and Transformation Fund has been, and remains, primarily focused on deficit reduction rather than transformation of services (Murray *et al* 2016b). The continuing use of the STF to sustain existing services was confirmed in the most recent NHS planning guidance (NHS England and NHS Improvement 2016a). A number of vanguard sites are reported to have scaled back their plans as a result of shortfalls in funding (Williams 2016).

The challenge is for national NHS bodies to see investment in new care models as part of the solution to achieving longer-term sustainability of NHS services. Doing this, of course, is far easier said than done; national leaders in the NHS themselves are under pressure from government to show how the NHS will fill growing gaps in finances and turn around declining performance. But the need for investment in new care models is inescapable in a context where existing services are struggling to meet the changing needs of the population. Part of the challenge for NHS leaders lies in making this case to the current government.

Ensure that the plans, and the assumptions underpinning them, are credible

The process for developing STPs described in this report has implications for the content of the plans and the confidence that should be placed in them. Most significantly, the speed at which they have been developed means that the details behind particular service changes often still need to be worked through – the exception being in areas where the STP is based on longer-term plans for redesigning services. Local leaders have also raised concerns about the assumptions underpinning financial projections made in their draft STPs. This is perhaps unsurprising – both because of the speed of the process, but also given the pressure from national NHS bodies to show how STPs will bring NHS finances back into balance, forcing leaders to look for radical solutions to reduce costs and improve efficiency.

Early analysis of draft STPs (Incisive Health 2016; Edwards 2016; Ham 2016) highlights the eye-watering efficiency assumptions that are often being made by local leaders. For example, many areas are seeking to make major reductions in the number of acute hospital beds by shifting care into primary and community settings. But there are reasons to be sceptical about whether these reductions can be delivered in the short term. A&E attendances and emergency admissions to hospital are on a rising trend (Murray *et al* 2016b). And growing pressures in general practice (Baird *et al* 2016), district nursing (Maybin *et al* 2016), mental health (Gilburt 2015) and social care services (Humphries *et al* 2016) mean that significant investment will be needed in services outside of hospitals if this shift in care is to be achieved. Even if it can be, the ability to make savings from these changes is by no means assured, depending on a range of factors, including whether fixed costs can be taken out of the system (Monitor 2015b).

This is not to say that ambitions to strengthen primary and community services and reduce demand for hospital care are wrong. It simply means that NHS leaders need to be realistic about what can be achieved within the timescales and levels of

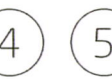   
funding available to them. It also means that final STPs will need to be 'stress-tested' to understand the assumptions behind plans for service changes and the benefits they are estimated to deliver. More honesty is needed about what can be delivered within the funding available to the NHS.

Focus on the skills and relationships needed to make STPs happen

The STP process so far has, unsurprisingly, focused on leaders working together to develop plans for the future of services in their area. But as the leaders involved in our research rightly pointed out, the real challenge lies in making these plans happen in practice. Doing this will require multiple changes made by staff from right across the health and care system – from teams working together to redesign care processes, to multiple organisations working together across large geographical areas to make improvements in specialist services like stroke or cancer care. Improvement will come from the aggregation of multiple changes made over time rather than single 'magic-bullet' solutions (Alderwick *et al* 2015b).

These kinds of changes will not happen by accident. They require intentional action on behalf of NHS leaders to equip staff with the skills and resources needed to make improvements in care (Ham *et al* 2016). They will also require far more attention to be placed on the cultural components of making change happen – including building trust and relationships – alongside the technical planning requirements that have played a major part in the STP process so far. We will explore these questions in more detail in the second part of our research, learning lessons from how our four STP footprints are approaching implementation of their plans.

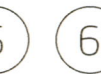

10 Conclusion

Our research has shown that the STP process so far has been far from perfect. It is important to recognise that our findings reflect the STP process up to July 2016, so do not include the final months of the planning process. Nonetheless, it is clear from our research that STPs have been developed at significant speed and without the meaningful involvement of frontline staff or the patients they serve. The plans are also being developed in an NHS policy environment that was not designed to support collaboration between organisations. But STPs are still in the early stages of development; in reality, the plans submitted in October 2016 represent the start of a longer-term process of improvement rather than the final word on how services will change. Lessons must be learnt from the weaknesses in the process so far. Changes to the statutory framework for the NHS may well be needed as the process develops. But collective action through STPs still offers a preferable alternative to the 'fortress mentality' whereby NHS organisations act to secure their own future regardless of the impact on others.

Summary of recommendations

- Involvement in the STP process should be strengthened at all levels within the health and care system, particularly among clinicians, frontline staff and local authorities.

- Meaningful involvement of patients and the public in the plans has not happened so far and must now be a priority.

- Governance arrangements that allow decisions to be made collectively between organisations and for accountability to be shared should be developed. Examples of where this is already happening should be shared across STP footprints.

- National bodies should remove the barriers that get in the way of local collaboration. NHS regulation, for example, must support collaboration between organisations rather than reinforcing divisions between them.

- National bodies in the NHS and the Department of Health should consider whether changes to the statutory framework for the NHS – for example, rules on competition and procurement – are needed to support collaboration through STPs.

- The role of named STP leaders should be clarified and strengthened – for example, by appointing full-time STP leaders and teams with dedicated resources to co-ordinate improvements in care.

- National bodies in the NHS should provide more co-ordinated leadership and support for STP footprints and the organisations within them. Better co-ordination is also needed between national and regional teams within NHS England and NHS Improvement.

- The STP process should be used to support the development of new models of care within the NHS and between the NHS and local government – not just the sustainability of existing services. Time and resources are needed to support this local transformation.

- National bodies in the NHS should 'stress-test' STPs to ensure that the assumptions underpinning them are credible and the changes they describe can be delivered. Realism is needed about what can be achieved within the timescales and funding available. Honesty is needed in communicating these messages to politicians and the public.

- National and local leaders should focus more attention on how STPs will be implemented. This will require intentional action on behalf of NHS leaders to create an environment that supports staff to make improvements in the services they deliver.

Appendix: STP timeline

Table 1 STP process timeline summary

Guidance, announcement or planning deadline	Date	Key points
NHS England, NHS Improvement, Health Education England, National Institute for Health and Care Excellence, Public Health England and Care Quality Commission publish *Delivering the Forward View: NHS planning guidance 2016/17–2020/21* (NHS England *et al* 2015; see also Alderwick and Ham 2016, McKenna and Dunn 2016)	22 December 2015	• Introduces the concept of STPs • NHS organisations are asked to produce two separate but connected plans – a one-year operational plan for 2016/17 (organisation-based) and a five-year STP (place-based) to deliver the aims of the Forward View • STPs are to cover 'all areas of CCG and NHS England commissioned activity' and 'must also cover better integration with local authority services' • An annex of indicative 'national challenges' sets out more than 60 questions to be addressed in the plans • STPs are to 'become the single application and approval process' for programmes with transformational funding for 2017/18, with the most compelling and credible securing the earliest additional funding • The first task for local health and care systems is to consider the geographic footprint for their STP, with proposals to NHS England by 29 January 2016, for national agreement • Submission of full STPs timetabled for end of June 2016, with assessment and review at the end of July 2016 • Further brief guidance on the STP process promised in January 2016
Monitor publishes paper on 'considerations for determining local health and care economies' (Monitor 2015a)	24 December 2015	• A piece of research and analysis from Monitor to 'help discussions' between local organisations for agreeing their STP footprints (identifies 37 local health and care economies)
Deadline for localities to submit proposals for STP footprints	29 January 2016	

continued on next page

Table 1 STP process timeline summary *continued*

Guidance, announcement or planning deadline	Date	Key points
STP guidance published by national NHS leaders (in the form of a letter) (NHS England 2016b)	16 February 2016	• Originally scheduled for publication at end of January • Introduces the idea that each footprint will have a nominated, named person responsible for 'overseeing and co-ordinating their STP process' – 'a senior and credible' leader who can command the trust and confidence of the system ('such as a CCG chief officer, provider chief executive or local authority chief executive'), with 'time and resource' expected to be dedicated • More detail to be published during the week of 29 February to help areas 'diagnose current and projected gaps'
Letter from Chair of LGA to Secretary of State for Health (Seccombe 2016)	10 March 2016	• Expresses support for STPs as 'a significant milestone in plotting the route to full integration of health and social care by 2020' • However, states 'concern' about the pace of implementation of STPs and the 'lack of consideration and involvement' of local councils in the process • Also expresses concern that footprints do not take account of the broader footprints for either existing or proposed combined authorities
44 geographical footprints announced (NHS England 2016h)	15 March 2016	• Average number of CCGs per footprint: 4.8 (range: 1–12) • Average footprint population: 1.2 million (range: 0.3 million–2.8 million) • The first eight STP leaders are also announced

STP leaders announced – in all but three areas (NHS England 2016g)	30 March 2016	• The leaders come from different organisations:
		  – 18 from CCGs
		  – 19 from NHS trusts or foundation trusts
		  – 3 from local government
		  – 1 already independent chair for the success regime
		  – 3 to be confirmed (later confirmed: 1 from local government; 1 interim lead from a CCG; 1 leadership consultant)

April STP checkpoint (NHS England 2016a)	15 April 2016	• Each STP makes a submission focusing on two questions: what leadership, decision-making processes and supporting resources have been put in place to make progress; and what are the major areas of focus and big decisions that will need to be made in each system to drive transformation

continued on next page

Table 1 **STP process timeline summary** *continued*

Guidance, announcement or planning deadline	Date	Key points
HSJ maps the financial health of every STP area (Dunhill 2016b)	22 April 2016	• Uses in-year financial performance by providers and CCGs in each STP to calculate each area's surplus or deficit as a proportion of turnover • Finds 'wide disparity' in the financial health of STPs • Identifies Cambridgeshire and Peterborough STP as 'the most challenging', with a combined deficit of around 13 per cent of turnover • Identifies Gloucester as the only STP area in which NHS organisations are reporting a combined surplus
One-to-one meetings with senior representatives from national NHS bodies	April/May 2016	
Health Education England agrees to regional team changes to support STPs (Health Education England 2016)	17 May 2016	• Including to create local workforce action boards (LWABs) to support and lead the workforce strand of STPs, and reducing the number of local education and training boards (LETBs) from 13 to 4 to align with the Forward View 'regional architecture'

Guidance on 30 June submission (now referred to as a 'checkpoint') sent to STP leaders (NHS England 2016f)	18 May 2016	• Submissions to include:
		  – shared understanding of where the STP is now in relation to the three gaps (health, quality and finance) and where they need to be by 2020/21
		  – the 'critical decisions' (priorities and transformation schemes) that will need to be made 'to shift the dial' and close the three gaps
		  – short-term and long-term delivery milestones
		  – financial template, showing how the STP will close financial gap in aggregate by 2020/21
		  – annexes covering governance and engagement and degree of consensus and support for changes
		• Plans will form basis of conversation with national NHS leadership in July

continued on next page

Table 1 **STP process timeline summary** *continued*

Guidance, announcement or planning deadline	Date	Key points
STPs are the subject of parliamentary questions for the first time (House of Commons 2016)	18 May 2016	• Three questions from Liberal Democrat MP Norman Lamb about: – STPs and mental health and integration of mental and physical health – engagement of communities, key stakeholders and voluntary and community sector – publication of STPs • Two questions from Green Party MP Caroline Lucas about: – the bodies involved in authorising STP footprints and the role of NHS Improvement – the definition of a system control total
Indicative funds to 2020 published (NHS England 2016c)	19 May 2016	• Following on from December 2015 publication of place-based funding allocations (comprising allocations for CCGs, primary and specialised services), this sets out indicative funding pots for all STP footprints to 2020/21 • Each STP allocation includes its share of the December 2015 allocations, plus its part of several national funding pots – including the Sustainability and Transformation Fund – divided up based on weighted capitation • Makes clear that STPs will be the 'single application and approval process' for being accepted onto programmes with transformational funding from 2017/18 onwards
'Quick guides' for STPs published by NHS England (2016d)	19 May 2016	• Two-page 'aides-mémoire' on a variety of topics to help local leaders work together in tackling the big system challenges. Fourteen topics covered, including cancer, prevention and new care models • Alongside the guides, national bodies offer a series of optional events designed to facilitate practical discussions about how to develop and deliver plans
Letter from NHS Improvement about seven-day services and STPs (NHS Improvement 2016b)	23 May 2016	• Unpublished letter to NHS Trust and Foundation Trust Medical Directors from NHS Improvement's Executive Medical Director, Dr Kathy McLean, setting out expectations for implementing seven-day services in light of developing STP plans

continued on next page

Table 1 STP process timeline summary *continued*

Guidance, announcement or planning deadline	Date	Key points
NHS Improvement publishes 'draft guidance on good governance in a local health economy' (NHS Improvement 2016a)	24 May 2016	• Sets out the additional standards of good governance that providers must meet when working collaboratively across local health and care economies • Reiterates that when collaborating, NHS providers 'must be mindful of the need to comply with their legal and regulatory obligations, for example in relation to choice and competition' • States that 'formal action' will be considered where providers are found not to be complying with standards

NHS England board paper on STPs (NHS England 2016j)	26 May 2016	• Provides update on STP review meetings taking place in May and June between each footprint and a national panel, consisting of Simon Stevens, at least two chief executives from national NHS bodies, the chief executive of the LGA and regional directors from NHS Improvement and NHS England
		• Provides 'reflections' from these meetings, including noting that:
		  – 'without exception, everyone welcomed the STP programme' as an 'incentive to seek system-based solutions to deep seated problems'
		  – STPs are at 'different starting points' and so the level of detail expected in June submissions will 'differ accordingly'
		  – there are 'lots of' good initiatives, but 'few yet at the degree of scale and pace required'
		  – workforce is a key issue 'in almost every footprint'
		  – there are 'impressive' partnerships with local authorities in many areas
		• STPs emphasised as 'means to deliver the vision set out in the Five Year Forward View' and as having 'galvanised the NHS'
		• Notes the need to be clear that 'this is not about "cutting" budgets, but about identifying the best possible use of resources so that we can meet the forecast rise in demand and, wherever possible, moderate that demand'

NHS England and NHS Improvement circulate a finance template to STP leads (NHS Improvement 2016d)	1 June 2016	• Asks each footprint to 'show how it will close its financial gap for NHS services and achieve sustainable financial balance in aggregate by 2020/21, with a focus on system-wide transformational solutions' • Ambulance providers serving multiple footprints are to submit an additional supplementary return to reflect the split of forecasted financial performance across footprints

continued on next page

Table 1 STP process timeline summary *continued*

Guidance, announcement or planning deadline	Date	Key points

NHS Confederation annual conference	17 June 2016	The topic of STPs is covered by many of the speakers, including:
		• Simon Stevens, Chief Executive of NHS England:
		  – 'to some extent these [STPs] are work-arounds on a set of institutional arrangements, a set of governance structures, and set of incentives that are pulling people apart, when actually we need to hang together'
		  – 'STPs… are a problem-solving process… a way of having a focused, honest, trusted conversation about some of the "elephants in the room", some of the "big ticket items", the difficult choices, that need to be resolved. How they are resolved will look different in different parts of the country. It is horses for courses'
		  – 'It is pretty obvious the money is not going to work if we carry on as we are'
		  – 'I wouldn't be surprised, if coming out of the STP process, we don't decide that in some places the local authorities might take on more of a leadership role for parts of, what have traditionally been, NHS functions'
		• Jeremy Hunt, Secretary of State for Health:
		  – 'The STPs are very simply about reducing hospital bed days per thousand population and reducing emergency admissions'

Letter from Jim Mackey and Ed Smith about the 2016/17 financial position (NHS England and NHS Improvement 2016b, Annex C)	28 June 2016	• Announces further action to bring down deficits. Areas asked to put together plans for pathology and back-office consolidation, and consolidation, change or transfer (to a neighbouring provider) of 'unsustainable' services • Asks STP leads to make proposals and identify relevant services by 31 July
Deadline for June 'checkpoint' submissions	30 June 2016	• NHS England FAQs (NHS England 2016i) says that 'we plan to publish Sustainability and Transformation Plans (STPs) once they are final', and regarding Freedom of Information requests states that 'As a result we expect that – subject to a public interest test – April submissions will exemption [sic] under section 22.'

continued on next page

Table 1 **STP process timeline summary** *continued*

Guidance, announcement or planning deadline	Date	Key points
Parliamentary questions relating to STPs	June 2016	• Eleven parliamentary questions asked about STPs in June, specifically concerning: – public access to STP meetings and notes and plans of meetings – public consultation on STP plans – the involvement of universities in the development of STPs – the legal status of STPs and the changes proposed – the identities of STP leaders – the 'accountability mechanics' for decision-making – the proportion of STPs submitted to the Department of Health – the deadlines for submission – the process for calculating place-based STP target allocations
Senior leaders within national NHS bodies visit all 44 STP areas	July 2016	• To review the draft STP submissions with each footprint • Conversations held throughout July between each of the 44 footprints and national NHS teams
Royal College of General Practitioners appoints 29 ambassadors (Twaddell 2016)	11 July 2016	• General practice ambassadors put in place to advance the GP Forward View and to represent general practice on STP boards
Simon Stevens appears before the Health Select Committee (House of Commons Health Committee 2016)	19 July 2016	• States that 'the majority of the country' will have 'well-designed service improvement and change plans come October' • Explains that although the plans are being developed locally, 'we see quite a lot of convergence'
Financial reset from NHS England and NHS Improvement (2016b)	21 July 2016	• States the intention to launch a two-year planning and contracting round , 'linked to agreed STPs', with joint planning guidance to be published in September • Gives further detail on implementation of the Lord Carter pathology and back-office consolidation (taking place at STP level) • Sets out the rules of operation for the 2016/17 Sustainability and Transformation Fund, which states that funding 'assumes full and effective participation in the STP process by each provider in receipt of an award' (although payment is not linked to STP engagement as was originally proposed) • Confirms that CCG allocation growth in 2017/18 is conditional on sign-off of STP • Final STP delivery plans are to be submitted in October

continued on next page

Table 1 STP process timeline summary *continued*

Guidance, announcement or planning deadline	Date	Key points
NHS England board paper on specialised commissioning (NHS England 2016e)	28 July 2016	• As part of work to align NHS England's 2017/18 commissioning intentions for specialised services with development of the 44 STP plans, NHS England states that it will be working with four STP areas (South East London, Herefordshire and Worcestershire, Greater Manchester and Cornwall) to demonstrate how specialised services can, within legal constraints, be integrated into place-based approaches to planning services
NHS Improvement writes to CEOs and finance directors of NHS trusts regarding plans to consolidate back-office and pathology services (Marlow and Warrington 2016)	July 2016	• Outlines the priority benchmark areas for STP business plans on back-office functions • States that a template for back-office and pathology have been created, which will be sent out to all providers in early September 2016, to be returned by the end of the month
Parliamentary questions relating to STPs	July 2016	• Five parliamentary questions asked about STPs, on: – STP plans for maternity services – the relationship between CCG transformation plans and STPs – the effect of STPs on geographical variations in stroke care – arrangements for consulting local authority members and the public
HSJ reports on an update from NHS England and NHS Improvement on final submissions (West 2016)	19 August 2016	• Specific formal feedback on draft plans given to each STP • Warns of an 'extremely constrained capital environment' and constraints on technology funding, encouraging STPs to explore 'other possible sources of funding' • System control totals to be made available to 'sufficiently advanced' STPs, although CCGs and NHS providers 'will remain accountable for their individual control totals' • Specifies that two-year planning guidance will be published on 20 September and that providers and CCGs will be expected to finalise two-year operational plans and contracts by end of December 2016 • Update on deadline for 'full' STP submissions (21 October 2016)

continued on next page

Table 1 STP process timeline summary *continued*

Guidance, announcement or planning deadline	Date	Key points
NHS Improvement publishes single oversight framework for NHS providers (NHS Improvement 2016c)	13 September 2016	• Sets out five themes, including 'strategic change'. NHS Improvement will 'consider how well providers are delivering the strategic changes set out in the 5YFV, with a particular focus on their contribution to sustainability and transformation plans (STPs), new care models, and, where relevant, implementation of devolution.'
An opposition day debate on STPs is held in the House of Commons	14 September 2016	• Labour motion, moved by Shadow Health Secretary Diane Abbott MP: 'That this House notes with concern that NHS Sustainability and Transformation Plans are expected to lead to significant cuts or changes to frontline services; believes that the process agreed by the Government in December 2015 lacks transparency and the timeline announced by NHS England is insufficient to finalise such a major restructure of the NHS; further believes that the timetable does not allow for adequate public or Parliamentary engagement in the formulation of the plans; and calls on the Government to publish the Plans and to provide an adequate consultation period for the public and practitioners to respond' • 50 MPs speak at the debate • The motion is rejected by the House (ayes: 195; noes: 280)

NHS England publishes guidance for involving patients and communities (NHS England *et al* 2016)	15 September 2016	• Guidance for teams developing STPs, intended to clarify the expectations on stakeholder involvement, in particular patient and public participation
		• Sets out expectations that:
		  – 'most areas' will take 'a version' of their STP to their organisation's public board meeting for discussion between late October and the end of the year
		  – 'most areas' will publish their plans, for more formal engagement, during this period

NHS England and NHS Improvement publish NHS operational planning and contracting guidance 2017–2019 *(continued on next page)*	22 September 2016	• Published in September rather than December to give organisations more time to plan and agree contracts 'earlier and for a longer duration' • For the first time, this planning guidance covers two financial years, with the default being for two-year contracts and a single NHS England and NHS Improvement oversight process to ensure alignment of CCG and provider plans

continued on next page

Table 1 STP process timeline summary *continued*

Guidance, announcement or planning deadline	Date	Key points
NHS England and NHS Improvement publish NHS operational planning and contracting guidance 2017–2019 (NHS England and NHS Improvement 2016a)	22 September 2016	• From April 2017, each STP to be given a financial control total (derived from individual control totals for CCGs and provider organisations in that geography) 'to ensure that organisational boundaries and perverse financial incentives do not get in the way of transformation'. It will be possible to 'flex' individual organisational control totals within the system control total 'by application', but the guidance states that two rules must be met: 'the provider sector achieves aggregate financial balance in 2017/18 and 2018/19, and the commissioning system continues to live within its statutory resource limits' • Included in the nine 2017/18 and 2018/19 'must dos' are requirements for STPs to implement agreed milestones, achieve agreed trajectories against STP core metrics, and achieve local system financial control totals • Sets out commitment to publish core baseline STP metrics in November 2016, 'drawing on existing data collections from the assurance frameworks'. This will include metrics on finance (specifically performance against control totals), quality (relating to A&E and referral to treatment (RTT) operational performance) and health outcomes and care redesign (for example, hospital total bed days per 1,000 population) • Sets a requirement for commissioner and provider plans to be aligned with their local STP's objectives and planning assumptions and demonstrate how they support delivery • Makes clear that operational plans for 2017/18 and 2018/19 are 'the detailed plans for the first two years of the STP' and that 'STP leaders will have strong governance processes' to ensure clarity as to how different organisations are 'contributing to agreed system working' • Announces that £1.8bn will be made available through the sustainability element of the Sustainability and Transformation Fund in 2017/18 and 2018/19, replicating arrangements in 2016/17, meaning little money will be left for transformation • States that the different streams of transformation funding available will 'increasingly be targeted towards the STPs making most progress' • Includes an annex setting out expectations for the content of STPs for the October 2016 submission (*see* below)

continued on next page

Table 1 STP process timeline summary *continued*

Guidance, announcement or planning deadline	Date	Key points

Parliamentary questions relating to STPs	September 2016	• Twenty-two parliamentary questions asked about STPs in September, on:
		  – discussions between the Department of Health and STP areas and publication of the minutes of these discussions
		  – public and local authority involvement in and consultation on the plans
		  – consultation of health and wellbeing boards and MPs on the plans
		  – publication of the plans
		  – cost of STPs
		  – public access to the feedback from NHS England to STP areas on the first drafts of their plans
		  – the number and cost of staff working on STPs (including in local and national NHS organisations as well as local authorities)
		  – the relationship between a specific contract and an STP
		  – various local STPs (including Staffordshire, West Sussex, Humber, Coast and Vale, Huddersfield and Calderdale CCG, Cheshire and Merseyside, Nottinghamshire, and South East London)
		  – discussions with the devolved administrations about STPs
		  – the inclusion of mobile surgical health centres
		  – parity of esteem between mental and physical health

HSJ reports on leaked guidance from NHS Improvement on financial control totals for 2017/18 and 2018/19 and STF allocations (Dunhill 2016a)	5 October 2016	• NHS Improvement issues guidance telling trusts they have until 24 November to agree new financial control totals for the next two years • The new control totals aim to bring the NHS provider sector into balance in 2017/18 • Trusts are required to agree their control total in order to receive their share of the STF • In 2017/18 the STF will 'again focus on supporting sustainability rather than transformation, aiming not to fund service enhancements but to sustain services'

continued on next page

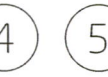
Table 1 STP process timeline summary *continued*

Guidance, announcement or planning deadline	Date	Key points
Deadline for final STP submissions (NHS England and NHS Improvement 2016a, Annex 4)	21 October 2016	• Plans expected to: – set out 'your plan to address the feedback from our July conversation' – provide 'more depth and specificity' on plans to implement the proposed schemes – set out a clear set of milestones, outcomes, resources and owners for each scheme, as well as overarching risks, governance and interdependencies – be underpinned by the finance template and show the impact on activity, benefits (costs and returns), capacity, workforce and investment requirements over time, building from a 'whole-system view developed in collaboration with local government colleagues' – set out the measurable impacts of the STP – set out the degree of local consensus among organisations and plans for further engagement • In addition, operational plans for individual CCGs and providers within an STP will be expected to reconcile to the STP
Other deadlines	24 November 2016	• Full draft operational plans for 2017/18 to 2018/19 to be submitted by CCGs and providers
	November 2016	• Feedback on October submissions from regional directors expected
	23 December 2016	• Target deadline for all 2017–19 contracts to be signed and final 2017/18 to 2018/19 operational plans (aligned with contracts) to be submitted by CCGs and providers

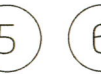 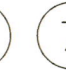

References

Alderwick H, Ham C (2016). 'The NHS in England embraces collaboration in tackling biggest crisis in its history'. *BMJ*, 352, i1022.

Alderwick H, Ham C, Buck D (2015a). *Population health systems: going beyond integrated care.* London: The King's Fund. Available at: www.kingsfund.org.uk/publications/population-health-systems (accessed on 19 October 2016).

Alderwick H, Robertson R, Appleby J, Dunn P, Maguire D (2015b). *Better value in the NHS: the role of changes in clinical practice.* London: The King's Fund. Available at: www.kingsfund.org.uk/publications/better-value-nhs (accessed on 19 October 2016).

Audit Commission (2005). *Governing partnerships: bridging the accountability gap.* London: Audit Commission. Available at: http://informationsharing.co.uk/wp-content/uploads/2012/08/Audit-commission-governing-partnerships.pdf (accessed on 19 October 2016).

Baird B, Charles A, Honeyman M, Maguire D, Das P (2016). *Understanding pressures in general practice.* London: The King's Fund. Available at: www.kingsfund.org.uk/publications/pressures-in-general-practice (accessed on 19 October 2016).

Bardsley M, Steventon A, Smith J, Dixon J (2013). *Evaluating integrated and community-based care: how do we know what works?* London: Nuffield Trust. Available at: www.nuffieldtrust.org.uk/publications/evaluating-integrated-and-community-based-care-how-do-we-know-what-works (accessed on 19 October 2016).

Collins B (2016). *New care models: emerging innovations in governance and organisational form.* London: The King's Fund. Available at: www.kingsfund.org.uk/publications/new-care-models (accessed on 19 October 2016).

Coulter A (2010). *Engaging communities for health improvement: a scoping study for the Health Foundation.* London: Health Foundation. Available at: www.health.org.uk/publication/engaging-communities-health-improvement (accessed on 19 October 2016).

Dunhill L (2016a). 'All trusts given new targets to achieve provider sector surplus'. *HSJ* website, 5 October.

Dunhill L (2016b). 'Mapped: the financial health of every STP area'. *HSJ* website, 22 April.

Dunn P, McKenna H, Murray R (2016). *Deficits in the NHS 2016.* London: The King's Fund. Available at: www.kingsfund.org.uk/publications/deficits-nhs-2016 (accessed on 19 October 2016).

Edwards N (2016). *Sustainability and transformation plans: what we know so far.* London: Nuffield Trust. Available at: www.nuffieldtrust.org.uk/publications/sustainability-and-transformation-plans-what-we-know-so-far (accessed on 19 October 2016).

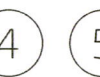
Everett A (2016). 'Warrington Borough Council chief executive Steven Broomhead says major reforms to town's health services are a "recipe for disaster"' [online]. *Warrington Guardian* website, 5 July. Available at: www.warringtonguardian.co.uk/news/14597299.Council_chief_executive_says_major_reforms_to_town_s_health_services_are_a__recipe_for_disaster_/ (accessed on 19 October 2016).

Foot C, Gilburt H, Dunn P, Jabbal J, Seale B, Goodrich J, Buck D, Taylor J (2014). *People in control of their own health and care: the state of involvement*. London: The King's Fund. Available at: www.kingsfund.org.uk/publications/people-control-their-own-health-and-care (accessed on 19 October 2016).

Gilburt H (2015). *Mental health under pressure*. London: The King's Fund. Available at: www.kingsfund.org.uk/publications/mental-health-under-pressure (accessed on 19 October 2016).

Ham C (2016). 'The need for a 45th STP – a national one'. *HSJ* website, 21 April.

Ham C (2014). *Reforming the NHS from within: beyond hierarchy, markets and inspection*. London: The King's Fund. Available at: www.kingsfund.org.uk/publications/reforming-nhs-within (accessed on 19 October 2016).

Ham C, Alderwick H (2015). *Place-based systems of care: a way forward for the NHS in England*. London: The King's Fund. Available at: www.kingsfund.org.uk/publications/place-based-systems-care (accessed on 19 October 2016).

Ham C, Baird B, Gregory S, Jabbal J, Alderwick H (2015). *The NHS under the coalition government: part one: NHS reform*. London: The King's Fund. Available at: www.kingsfund.org.uk/publications/nhs-under-coalition-government (accessed on 26 October 2016).

Ham C, Berwick D, Dixon J (2016). *Improving quality in the NHS in England: a strategy for action*. London: The King's Fund. Available at: www.kingsfund.org.uk/publications/quality-improvement (accessed on 19 October 2016).

Hansard (House of Commons Debates) (2016–17) 14 September 2016 col 949. Available at: http://hansard.parliament.uk/commons/2016-09-14/debates/16091433000002/NHSSustainability AndTransformationPlans (accessed on 19 October 2016).

Health Education England (2016). *Agenda for board meeting 17 May 2016, item 9: Health Education England, delivering the five year forward view* [online]. Health Education England website. Available at: https://hee.nhs.uk/about-us/our-leaders-structure/hee-board/board-meetings-papers/hee-board-meeting-17-may-2016 (accessed on 19 October 2016).

Health Foundation, The King's Fund (2015). *Making change possible: a transformation fund for the NHS*. London: Health Foundation and The King's Fund. Available at: www.kingsfund.org.uk/publications/making-change-possible (accessed on 19 October 2016).

House of Commons (2016). 'Written questions and answers' [online]. Available at: www.parliament.uk/business/publications/written-questions-answers-statements/written-questions-answers/?page=1&max=20&questiontype=AllQuestions&house=commons%2Clords&member=1439&dept=17&keywords=Mental%2CHealth (accessed on 19 October 2016).

House of Commons Health Committee (2016). *Oral evidence: NHS current issues 2016*. HC 299. Available at: www.parliament.uk/business/committees/committees-a-z/commons-select/health-committee/inquiries/parliament-2015/nhs-england-current-issues-one-off-evidence-16-17/publications/ (accessed on 19 October 2016).

House of Commons Public Accounts Committee (2016). *Oral evidence: UnitingCare Partnership contract*. HC 633. Available at: www.parliament.uk/business/committees/committees-a-z/commons-select/public-accounts-committee/inquiries/parliament-2015/unitingcare-partnership-contract-16-17/publications/ (accessed on 19 October 2016).

Humphries R, Thorlby R, Holder H, Hall P, Charles A (2016). *Social care for older people: home truths*. London: The King's Fund. Available at: www.kingsfund.org.uk/publications/social-care-older-people (accessed on 19 October 2016).

Imison C, Sonola L, Honeyman M, Ross S (2014). *The reconfiguration of clinical services: what is the evidence?* London: The King's Fund. Available at: www.kingsfund.org.uk/publications/reconfiguration-clinical-services (accessed on 19 October 2016).

Incisive Health (2016). *STPs: early areas of action*. Available at: www.incisivehealth.com/uploads/images/services/38%20Degrees%20-%20STP%20Early%20Action%20Report%20-%20August%202016.pdf (accessed on 19 October 2016).

Marlow and Warrington (2016). 'Consolidation of back office and pathology services'. *Provider Bulletin*, 17 August. NHS Improvement website. Available at: https://improvement.nhs.uk/news-alerts/provider-bulletin-17-august-2016/#pathology (accessed on November 4 2016).

Maybin J, Charles A, Honeyman M (2016). *Understanding quality in district nursing services: learning from patients, carers and staff*. London: The King's Fund. Available at: www.kingsfund.org.uk/publications/quality-district-nursing (accessed on 19 October 2016).

McKenna H, Dunn P (2016). *What the planning guidance means for the NHS: 2016/17 and beyond*. London: The King's Fund. Available at: www.kingsfund.org.uk/publications/what-planning-guidance-means-nhs (accessed on 29 September 2016).

Monitor (2015a). *Considerations for determining local health and care economies* [online]. GOV.UK website. Available at: www.gov.uk/government/publications/considerations-for-determining-local-health-and-care-economies (accessed on 19 October 2016).

Monitor (2015b). 'Moving healthcare closer to home'. GOV.UK website. Available at: www.gov.uk/guidance/moving-healthcare-closer-to-home (accessed on 19 October 2016).

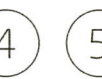

Murray R, Edwards N, Imison C (2016a). 'Don't rush to reconfigure: there is another way'. *HSJ* website, 29 July.

Murray R, Jabbal J, Thompson J, Maguire D (2016b). 'How is the NHS performing? Quarterly monitoring report 20'. The King's Fund website. Available at: http://qmr.kingsfund.org.uk/2016/20/ (accessed on 19 October 2016).

Mulley A, Trimble C, Elwyn G (2012). *Patients' preferences matter: stop the silent misdiagnosis.* London: The King's Fund. Available at: www.kingsfund.org.uk/publications/patients-preferences-matter (accessed on 19 October 2016).

Naylor C, Das P, Ross S, Honeyman M, Thompson J, Gilburt H (2016). *Bringing together physical and mental health: a new frontier for integrated care.* London: The King's Fund. Available at: www.kingsfund.org.uk/publications/physical-and-mental-health (accessed on 19 October 2016).

NHS England (2016a). *Developing sustainability and transformation plans: preparing for 15 April and beyond* [online]. Slideset. Available at: www.local.gov.uk/integration-better-care-fund/-/journal_content/56/10180/7772969/ARTICLE (accessed on 19 October 2016).

NHS England (2016b). 'Developing sustainability and transformation plans to 2020/21'. Letter. Available at: www.england.nhs.uk/wp-content/uploads/2016/02/sustainability-transformation-plan-letter-160216.pdf (accessed on 20 October 2016).

NHS England (2016c). 'NHS England sets out local NHS funding growth to 2020'. NHS England website. Available at: www.england.nhs.uk/2016/05/local-funding-growth-to-2020/ (accessed on 19 October 2016).

NHS England (2016d). 'Quick guides: May 2016'. NHS England website. Available at: www.england.nhs.uk/ourwork/futurenhs/deliver-forward-view/stp/support/ (accessed on 19 October 2016).

NHS England (2016e). *Specialised Services Commissioning Committee (SSCC) report to board* [online]. NHS England Board meeting papers, 28 July, item 13.iii. NHS England website. Available at: www.england.nhs.uk/2016/07/board-meet-28-july-16/ (accessed on 19 October 2016.

NHS England (2016f). 'STP 30th June submission' [online]. NHS England website. Available at: www.england.nhs.uk/wp-content/uploads/2016/05/stp-submission-guidance-june.pdf (accessed on 19 October 2016).

NHS England (2016g). 'Sustainability and Transformation leaders confirmed'. NHS England website. Available at: www.england.nhs.uk/2016/03/leaders-confirmed/ (accessed on 20 October 2016).

NHS England (2016h). *Sustainability and Transformation Plan footprints* [online]. NHS England website. Available at: www.england.nhs.uk/wp-content/uploads/2016/02/stp-footprints-march-2016.pdf (accessed on 19 October 2016).

NHS England (2016i). *Sustainability and Transformation Plans* [online]. Slideset. Available at: www.qehkl.nhs.uk/Documents/STP%20QA%20June%202016%2020160615.pdf (accessed on 19 October 2016).

NHS England (2016j). *Sustainability and Transformation Plans: progress and next steps* [online]. NHS England board meeting papers, 26 May. NHS England website. Available at: www.england.nhs.uk/2016/05/board-meet-26-may-16/ (accessed on 19 October 2016).

NHS England (2016k). 'We need patients and the public to shape local health plans, say NHS leaders'. NHS England website. Available at: www.england.nhs.uk/2016/09/local-health-plans/ (accessed on 20 October 2016).

NHS England, NHS Improvement (2016a). *NHS shared planning guidance: NHS operational planning and contracting guidance 2017–2019*. NHS England website. Available at: www.england.nhs.uk/ourwork/futurenhs/deliver-forward-view/ (accessed on 19 October 2016).

NHS England, NHS Improvement (2016b). *Strengthening financial performance and accountability in 2016/17* [online]. NHS England website. Available at: www.england.nhs.uk/publications/performance/ (accessed on 19 October 2016).

NHS England, NHS Improvement, Health Education England, National Institute for Health and Care Excellence, Public Health England, Care Quality Commission (2016). *Engaging local people: a guide for local areas developing Sustainability and Transformation Plans*. NHS England website. Available at: www.england.nhs.uk/ourwork/futurenhs/deliver-forward-view/stp/support/#localstp (accessed on 19 October 2016).

NHS England, NHS Improvement, Health Education England, National Institute for Health and Care Excellence, Public Health England, Care Quality Commission (2015). *Delivering the Forward View: NHS planning guidance 2016/17–2020/21*. NHS England website. Available at: www.england.nhs.uk/ourwork/futurenhs/deliver-forward-view/ (accessed on 19 October 2016).

NHS England, Public Health England (2013). *A call to action: commissioning for prevention*. NHS England website. Available at: www.england.nhs.uk/ourwork/qual-clin-lead/calltoaction/ (accessed on 19 October 2016).

NHS Improvement (2016a). *Guidance for providers on good governance in local health economy working* [online]. NHS Improvement website. Available at: https://improvement.nhs.uk/resources/draft-guidance-good-governance-local-health-economy/ (accessed on 19 October 2016).

NHS Improvement (2016b). 'How can seven day services benefit patients?' [online]. *Provider bulletin*, 25 May. NHS Improvement website. Available at: https://improvement.nhs.uk/news-alerts/provider-bulletin-25-may-2016/#seven (accessed on 20 October 2016).

NHS Improvement (2016c). *Single oversight framework*. NHS Improvement website. Available at: https://improvement.nhs.uk/resources/single-oversight-framework/ (accessed on 19 October 2016).

NHS Improvement (2016d). 'Sustainability and Transformation Plans: finance and efficiency template released' [online]. NHS Improvement website. Available at: https://improvement.nhs.uk/news-alerts/provider-bulletin-8-june-2016/#template (accessed on 20 October 2016).

Oliver D, Foot C, Humphries R (2014). *Making our health and care systems fit for an ageing population*. London: The King's Fund. Available at: www.kingsfund.org.uk/publications/making-our-health-and-care-systems-fit-ageing-population (accessed on 19 October 2016).

Ostrom E (2010). 'Beyond markets and states: polycentric governance of complex economic systems'. *American Economic Review*, vol 100, no 3, pp 641–72.

Ostrom E (1990). *Governing the commons: the evolution of institutions for collective action*. Cambridge: Cambridge University Press.

Sandford M (2016). *Combined authorities* [online]. Briefing paper number 06649. House of Commons Library website. Available at: http://researchbriefings.parliament.uk/ResearchBriefing/Summary/SN06649#fullreport (accessed on 19 October 2016).

Seccombe I (2016). 'Letter from Cllr Izzi Seccombe to Jeremy Hunt on STPs'. Local Government Association website. Available at: www.local.gov.uk/integration-better-care-fund/-/journal_content/56/10180/7772969/ARTICLE (accessed on 19 October 2016).

Senge P, Hamilton H, Kania J (2015). 'The dawn of system leadership'. Stanford Social Innovation Review website. Available at: https://ssir.org/articles/entry/the_dawn_of_system_leadership#bio-footer (accessed on 19 October 2016).

Steventon A, Bardsley M, Billings J, Georghiou T, Lewis G (2011). *An evaluation of the impact of community-based interventions on hospital use*. London: Nuffield Trust. Available at: www.nuffieldtrust.org.uk/publications/evaluation-impact-community-based-interventions-hospital-use (accessed on 19 October 2016).

Timmins N (2015). *The practice of system leadership: being comfortable with chaos*. London: The King's Fund. Available at: www.kingsfund.org.uk/publications/practice-system-leadership (accessed on 19 October 2016).

Twaddell I (2016). 'RCGP appoints 29 GP "ambassadors" to advance Forward View'. *Pulse* website, 11 July.

West D (2016). 'Exclusive: officials warn over "extremely constrained" capital for STPs'. *HSJ* website, 25 August.

Williams D (2016). 'Exclusive: vanguards scale back plans due to funding shortfall'. *HSJ* website, 20 September.

Wilson S, Davison N, Clarke M, Casebourne J (2015). *Joining up public services around local, citizen needs: perennial challenges and insights on how to tackle them*. London: Institute for Government. Available at: www.instituteforgovernment.org.uk/publications/joining-up-local-services (accessed on 19 October 2016).

Wilkinson J, Powell A, Davies H (2011). *Are clinicians engaged in quality improvement? A review of the literature on healthcare professionals' view on quality improvement initiatives*. London: Health Foundation. Available at: www.health.org.uk/publication/are-clinicians-engaged-quality-improvement (accessed on 19 October 2016).

About the authors

Hugh Alderwick is Senior Policy Adviser to Chris Ham. Since joining The King's Fund in 2014, Hugh has published work on NHS reform, integrated care and population health, and opportunities for the NHS to improve value for money. Before joining the Fund, Hugh worked as a management consultant in PricewaterhouseCoopers' (PwC) health team.

Hugh was seconded from PwC to work on Sir John Oldham's Independent Commission on Whole Person Care, which reported to the Labour Party at the beginning of 2014. The Commission looked at how health and care services can be more closely aligned to deliver integrated services meeting the whole of people's needs.

Phoebe Dunn is a researcher in the policy team, primarily working to help the wider team stay on top of the changing policy environment, as well as contributing to a range of health and care research projects.

Before joining the Fund, Phoebe worked for a marketing and strategy agency on projects for small and large organisations from across the health and care sector. These included the launch report for the Point of Care Foundation, digital strategy for a large health charity, and a myth-busting campaign around outcomes-based approaches to health care.

Helen McKenna is a generalist whose role spans The King's Fund's policy and communications functions and involves identifying, analysing and communicating emerging policy issues as well as advising on their implications.

Before joining the Fund, Helen worked as principal policy adviser on health and social care at Which? and as a fast-stream trainee and then manager at the Department of Health. Her roles at the Department included working on the Health and Social Care Act reforms, leading a review of the NHS Constitution and developing a programme of collaboration on health matters between China and the UK.

Helen has an MSc in health policy from Imperial College London.

Nicola Walsh is Assistant Director of Leadership and Organisational Development at The King's Fund and leads its cross-fund programme on integrated care.

She was a director in the health consulting practice at PwC for five years before joining the Fund in 2012. She has worked in and with the NHS for more than 25 years, first as a clinician, then as a researcher at the Centre of Health Economics in York and at the University of Birmingham, and more recently as a non-executive director.

Nicola has a Masters degree in health policy and management and a PhD in health services research. She is a trustee of a national charity, the Queen's Nursing Institute, and has recently been appointed a member of an expert advisory group set up by the Royal Pharmaceutical Society to look into future models of care.

Chris Ham leads The King's Fund's work. He rejoined the Fund in 2010, having previously worked for the organisation between 1986 and 1992. He has held posts at the universities of Birmingham, Bristol and Leeds and is currently emeritus professor at the University of Birmingham. He is an honorary fellow of the Royal College of Physicians of London and the Royal College of General Practitioners.

Chris was director of the strategy unit in the Department of Health between 2000 and 2004, has advised the World Health Organization and the World Bank, and has acted as a consultant to a number of governments. He has been a non-executive director of the Heart of England NHS Foundation Trust, and a governor of the Health Foundation and the Canadian Health Services Research Foundation.

Chris researches and writes on all aspects of health reform and is a sought-after speaker. He was awarded a CBE in 2004 for his services to the NHS and an honorary doctorate by the University of Kent in 2012.

Acknowledgements

We would like to thank everyone in the four STP areas who took part in our interviews. We are grateful for their time – particularly given our findings about the strain of the STP process. We would particularly like to thank the STP leaders in these four areas for their support throughout the research and their comments on the draft report.

We would also like to thank colleagues at The King's Fund for reviewing the draft report and helping to co-ordinate the research and Clare Sutherland for her help in arranging site visits and interviews.

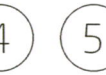
Published by
The King's Fund
11–13 Cavendish Square
London W1G 0AN
Tel: 020 7307 2568
Fax: 020 7307 2801

Email:
publications@kingsfund.org.uk

www.kingsfund.org.uk

© The King's Fund 2016

First published 2016 by
The King's Fund

Charity registration number:
1126980

All rights reserved, including
the right of reproduction in
whole or in part in any form

ISBN: 978 1 909029 69 9

A catalogue record for this
publication is available from
the British Library

Edited by Kathryn O'Neill

Typeset by
Grasshopper Design Company

Printed in the UK by
The King's Fund

The King's Fund is an independent charity working to improve health and care in England. We help to shape policy and practice through research and analysis; develop individuals, teams and organisations; promote understanding of the health and social care system; and bring people together to learn, share knowledge and debate. Our vision is that the best possible care is available to all.

www.kingsfund.org.uk @thekingsfund